Future of Cardiovascular Health

Mohamed Shalaby, MD

ISBN: 1981744290
ISBN 13: 9781981744299

Publication Details

No part of this publication may be reproduced, stored in a retrieval system, or transmitted in any form or by any means, electronic, mechanical, photocopying, recording, scanning, or otherwise, except as permitted under Sections 107 or 108 of the 1976 United States Copyright Act, without the prior written permission of the author. Requests to the author for permission should be addressed online at drshalaby@txheartcenter.com.

To my patients; thank you for the privilege of being your doctor. You have taught me so much about life and medicine.

I would like to express my gratitude to the many people who helped me through this book. To Dina and the children and to my colleagues and friends who provided support and feedback throughout the process of creating this book.

Contents

Preface

This book, *Future of Cardiovascular Health*, highlights technological contributions to the treatment of cardiovascular diseases. This book is one key to understanding how technology is the future of health care and exercise. The revolutionary concepts introduced herein will change the way we evaluate and treat cardiac disease now and in the future. This book takes a holistic approach to cardiovascular care while highlighting the influence of social media, digital technology, genetic modifications, meditation, spiritual practices, exercise, minimally invasive procedures, with a focus on technological innovations.

Chapter 1

How Did We Get Here?

1.1 Overview

The term "cardiovascular disease" (often abbreviated to CVD) refers to the negative conditions that affect the heart or blood vessels. In medical circles, cardiovascular disease is also known as circulatory or heart disease but it is not a single disease; rather, it is a cluster of diseases, many of which are related to atherosclerosis or the build up of plaque on the walls of the arteries. When plaque builds up, it causes the arteries to narrow, which constricts the normal flow of blood. This leads to an increased risk of blood clots, which causes damage to crucial organs such as the brain, kidney, heart, and eyes. All forms of CVD combined are the leading cause of death globally and people aged between thirty and forty-four are more vulnerable to CVD. However, most cardiologists believe that those who develop a form of cardiovascular disease around the age of thirty-five already show the initial symptoms of this disease.

1.1.1 Types of Cardiovascular Diseases

The various types of CVD include the following:

- ❖ Coronary heart disease (CHD)
  CHD is also known as atherosclerotic heart disease or coronary artery disease (CAD). This form of CVD is caused by the buildup of athermatous plaques within the walls of the arteries that supply blood to the heart muscle. CHD symptoms arise in advanced stages with most individuals who have the disease being unaware of it until these symptoms present. A sudden heart attack is often the first symptom of CHD.

- ❖ Angina
  Angina is chest discomfort associated with advanced coronary heart disease. The discomfort can occur in various forms, such as pressure or squeezing in the chest, pain in the jaw, arm, and so on. Angina varies in intensity with most individuals not experiencing much pain. Essentially, the discomfort is a result of a cramp in the heart muscle.

- ❖ Rheumatic heart disease (RHD)
  Rheumatic heart disease is preventable and treatable. RHD is a form of CVD wherein the aortic valve or mitral valve is permanently damaged. Both valves are sometimes damaged by rheumatic fever as a result of streptococcal infection. Rheumatic fever is an inflammatory disease that affects connective tissues in the body, especially those of the joints, brain, and heart. The fever is rampant in children between the ages of five and fifteen. RHD symptoms can linger in individuals for life or reappear ten to twenty years after the original appearance of the disease. In the heart, the mitral valve is more prone to the disease than the aortic valve.

- ❖ Stroke
  Stroke is an acute neurological injury that results when the blood supply to a part of the brain is interrupted or reduced. This happens largely because of an arterial rupture (also known as a hemorrhage) or blockage. The part of the brain affected receives little or no oxygen, therefore the cells in that part of the brain die or become damaged, which impairs brain function. If not promptly diagnosed or treated, stroke can cause permanent neurological damage or death.

- ❖ Congenital heart disease

Congenital heart disease is a general term used to describe multiple abnormalities that affect the heart. These abnormalities are primarily due to an abnormal development of the heart occurring before birth. In some cases, like the coarctation or narrowing of the aorta, it is possible for one to live with the abnormality without any alarm. Additionally, lesions like a small ventricular septal defect cause no problems and allow a person with this defect to live a normal life and engage in normal physical activity.

❖ Peripheral arterial disease
This is a circulatory problem caused by narrowed peripheral arteries. The narrowing occurs when plaque accumulates in arteries, causing a reduced blood flow to the limbs. Peripheral arterial disease can also involve an accumulation of large amounts of fat in the arteries, causing reduced blood flow to the legs, brain, heart, and other body parts. This disease is characterized by pain and numbness in the limbs.

❖ Aortic aneurysm and dissections
This form of cardiovascular disease occurs when an artery inflates like a balloon. An aneurysm occurs in parts of the aorta, the left ventricle, and arteries that supply blood to the brain. This happens when an artery wall is torn or separation of an artery wall's layers allows for a flow of blood between them. This hinders free movement of blood, causing the aneurysm to burst.

❖ Deep vein thrombosis
This condition occurs when a blood clot develops in the deep veins. Frequently, deep vein thrombosis happens when one has a medical condition that affects normal blood clotting in the body such as prolonged bed rest, pregnancy, smoking, obesity, surgery, or cancer. Deep vein thrombosis is associated with life-threatening

pulmonary embolism, which is characterized by coughing up blood, shortness of breath, rapid pulse, and dizziness. This condition damages the veins and reduces blood flow to the affected areas.

❖ Cardiomyopathy (heart muscle disorder)
Cardiomyopathy is a condition involving an abnormal heart muscle. A heart with cardiomyopathy means that the heart is unable to adequately pump blood to the rest of the body. Cardiomyopathy is sometimes inherited; at other times it can be caused by heart attacks or viral infections.

❖ Heart valve disorders and diseases
A heart valve disorder occurs when a heart valve does not adequately perform its functions. Heart valves are located at each exit of the heart chamber. They ensure the free forward flow of blood without backward leakage. These disorders are caused by age, infections, heart attack, hypertension; they can also be congenital. Heart valve disease is characterized by dizziness, chest discomfort, palpitations, swelling in the ankles and feet, difficulty breathing, and rapid weight gain.

1.2 The Burden

The prevalence of cardiovascular disease is difficult to estimate since many cases go undiagnosed. Also, patients' lack of seriousness toward their health makes it impossible to prevent cardiovascular disease. Countries report the prevalence of cardiovascular disease in different ways making it difficult to ascertain an accurate number. While we will consider data from across the globe, we will focus primarily on the United States as an example, and take a look at the alarming statistics of cardiovascular disease.

According to a report from the American Heart Association (2015 update), data from more than 190 countries shows that

CVD remains the single leading cause of death globally accounting for over 17.3 million deaths annually. According to this report, that number is projected to increase to more than 23.6 million deaths by 2030. Stroke is the second leading cause of death. In 2010, thirty-three million people experienced first or recurrent strokes.

In 2013, CVD accounted for 31 percent of total global deaths. In the United States, 801,000 deaths every year were due to CVD, meaning about one out of three people who die did so as a result of CVD. CVD accounts for about 2,200 deaths a day; or an average of one death every forty seconds. Moreover, 19.2 million American adults live with some form of CVD or the aftereffects of stroke. According to the American Heart Association, CVD accounts for around 45.1 percent of deaths in the United States; stroke for 16.5 percent; heart failure, 8.5 percent; high blood pressure, 9.1 percent; artery diseases, 3.2 percent; and the other assorted CVDs for the remaining 7.8 percent of CVD deaths in the United States.

1.2.1 Geographic Spread

The main causes of cardiovascular disease in the United Kingdom and the United States, both developed countries, are obesity, lack of exercise, and poor diet. Eighteen percent of the total daily death rate in high-income countries is caused by CVD. This figure is reduced to 10 percent in low- and middle-income nations. Stroke is recorded as a leading cause of all the major disabilities in the United Kingdom.

People living in undeveloped countries have a higher risk of CVD than those living in well-developed countries. Over 60 percent of the global CHD burden is in developing countries. The largest CHD death tolls have been recorded in Russia, China, and India. Similar figures for stroke fatalities have also been exhibited by developing countries.

The treatment of CVD in developed countries has improved considerably over the last ten years. As a result, mortality in developed countries has gradually decreased. As the developed world makes strides towards prevention and treatment of CVDs, it is predicted that the rates of CVD in developing countries will drop accordingly. However, there is still serious concern about CVD in developing nations. As the prevalence of the major risk factors for CVD (including diabetes and obesity) increase, we can expect a corresponding rise in the prevalence of CVD. Studies predict that in 2025, over 140 million people will be suffering from diabetes or obesity, making them prime candidates for CVD. In short, while treatments are improving and rates of prevention are increasing, risk factors are increasing as well. As countries develop and wealth increases, CVD risk factors also increase.

1.2.2 Economic and Socioeconomic Costs

The economic costs associated with cardiovascular disease are vast and include health-care, loss of productivity, and general care costs. The economic costs of CVD are substantial in countries with a high morbidity rate due to stroke and CHD. In 2010, the global economic cost of CVD was estimated at $863 billion. This number is predicted to increase to over one billion dollars by 2030. According to the National Heart, Lung, and Blood Institute, the cost of cardiovascular disease in the United States alone for 2006 was $400 billion, nearly half the global total. The figure is expected to rise meteorically, with the World Health Organization (WHO) estimating the cost will increase by a whopping 25 percent in 2030.

1.3 Risk Factors

Although cardiovascular disease is a complex class of multiple conditions, the risk factors are well known. They include:

- ❖ smoking
- ❖ obesity
- ❖ diabetes
- ❖ high blood pressure
- ❖ high LDL cholesterol
- ❖ social, economic risks

These risk factors can interact with and affect each other, adding to the medical complications presented by the disease. For example, obesity can increase the risk for diabetes, which subsequently increases the risk for CVD. As a result, it is virtually impossible to establish a comprehensive method of predicting CVD based on risk factors. Additionally, having multiple risk factors increases a person's probability of contracting CVD.

1.4 History and Timelines

The first cardiovascular research was conducted in China in the twenty-sixth century BC when Huang Ti deduced that blood flows in a circulatory system with the heart as the engine.[1] Over the years, advances by individuals such as Leonardo da Vinci (fifteenth century), have also been recorded. Da Vinci described atherosclerosis but did not coin the term (WHO). It wasn't until the nineteenth century that real-paced research on the cardiovascular system took off, thanks to the discovery of cholesterol, the electrical pulse of the heartbeat, and the description of atherosclerotic plaque. Modern clinical cardiology relies heavily on major discoveries of the twentieth century. One of the biggest steps forward in both treatment and prevention has been the implementation of electrical devices and implants. Implanting electrical devices like pacemakers that monitor the heart's electrical activity is one example of the integration of technology into cardiology.

---

[1] World Health Organization's 2004 journal, *Atlas of Heart Disease and Stroke.*

What follows is a chronology of key events in cardiology from 1856 to present day[2]:

❖ 1856: Rudolf Virchow, a German pathologist, biologist, and prehistorian, believed that cardiovascular disease occurred at the cellular level. He described how cerebral emboli caused strokes and emphasized the effects of societal issues on heart diseases.

❖ 1867: An English pharmacologist named Lauder Brunton discovered that amyl nitrate cured angina.

❖ 1872: Franco-Luxembourgish physician and inventor Gabriel Lippmann invented the capillary electrometer, a precursor to the electrocardiograph.

❖ 1893: Willem Einthoven of the Netherlands coined the name "electrocardiogram" (also known as the ECG or EKG) and distinguished its five deflections.

❖ 1895: Wilhelm Conrad Roentgen of Germany discovered the x-rays used in the visualization of the human heart.

❖ 1896: Scipione Riva of Italy invented the sphygmomanometer to help measure blood pressure.

❖ 1897: Modern aspirin was introduced. The first aspirin developed by Bayer was advertised as a drug that caused no effect to the human heart.

❖ 1906: Matthias Cremer of Germany invented the first esophageal ECG besides the fetal EKG/ECG for the lower surface of pregnant women's bodies.

❖ 1907: Arthur Cushy of England, a pharmacology professor, reported the first case of atrial fibrillation.

❖ 1912: The first cardiac catheterization with no x-ray visualization was performed by Ernst Unger, Fritz Bleichroeder, and Werner Loeb.

❖ 1915: The American Heart Association was established in the United States in New York.

---

[2] World Health Organization's *Atlas of Heart Disease and Stroke*.

- ❖ 1920: Harold Pardee, an American cardiologist, performed the first ECG of an acute myocardial infarction.
- ❖ 1923: Americans Samuel A. Levine and Elliott Carr Cutler performed the first operation to widen a damaged cardiac valve.
- ❖ 1925: In the United Kingdom, a surgeon widened a narrowed mitral valve using fingers.
- ❖ 1928: Sir Alexander Fleming discovered penicillin in the United Kingdom.
- ❖ 1928: The term "apoplexy" was replaced by "cerebral vascular accident."
- ❖ 1929: Werner Forssmann of Germany performed the first right heart catheterization using radiographic techniques.
- ❖ 1931: Charles Wolferth and Francis Wood of the United States described the importance of exercise in provoking angina pectoris attacks.
- ❖ 1931: Dr. Albert Hyman of the United States used an artificial cardiac pacemaker to stimulate the heart with a transthoracic needle.
- ❖ 1937: American John Heysham Gibbon built the first prototype heart-lung machine which would be used to perform the first open-heart operation in 1953.
- ❖ 1938: American surgeon Dr. Robert E. Gross performed the first known surgical correction of a congenital heart defect.
- ❖ 1944: The first corrective operation of the caucus arteries was performed in China. In the same year, doctors at John Hopkins Hospital in the United States performed an operation to correct blue baby syndrome (Fallot's tetralogy). During the same year, Balcarras Crafoord and Berthold Grosse performed the first aorta repair in Sweden.
- ❖ 1947: Dr. Charles Bailey and Dr. Dwight Harken, both of the United States, performed the first closed surgery of a mitral stenosis.

- ❖ 1948: Lawrence Craven, an American physician based in California, discovered that four hundred male patients who took aspirin for two years suffered no heart attacks. By 1956, Craven registered over eight thousand people taking aspirin who suffered no heart attacks.
- ❖ 1949: In the United States, the Framingham Heart Study began and many healthy men and women were studied. In the same year, Norman Holter invented the first portable Holter monitor to record ambulatory EKGs.
- ❖ 1950: The International Society of Cardiology was founded. This organization later joined the International Cardiology Federation to form the World Heart Federation. Later in 1950, John Hopps of Canada invented the first pacemaker.
- ❖ 1952: In the United States, a prosthetic valve was implanted in the aorta for the first time by surgeon Charles Hufnagel. Also in that year, Clarence Walton Lillehei and Floyd John Lewis performed the first successful open-heart operation under hypothermia. They successfully implanted a synthetic valve in the heart of a five-year-old girl who had been born with a hole in her heart. In that same year, the first external cardiac pacemaker was designed by Paul Zoll.
- ❖ 1953: Coronary heart disease was first reported among American soldiers killed in action in Korea during the Korean War.
- ❖ 1954: H. H. G. Eastcott, G. W. Pickering, and C. G. Rob performed a carotid endarterectomy in the United Kingdom. During the same year, India urged the World Health Organization to look into the alarming rates of cardiovascular disease recorded in third-world countries.
- ❖ 1955: Judson Chesterman of the United Kingdom performed the first mitral valve replacement.

- ❖ 1955: The introduction of randomization was made in clinical trials to minimize bias in the assessment of cardiovascular disease treatments.
- ❖ 1956: Dr. Paul Zoll of the United States published the first successful correction of ventricular fibrillation by external application of a countershock.
- ❖ 1957: The first introduction of an external pacemaker powered by a battery was recorded.
- ❖ 1958: Dr. Ake Senning of Sweden introduced an internal long-term cardiac pacemaker. That same year in the United States, Dr. Seymour Furman successfully inserted an artificial pacemaker into a patient who survived for ninety-six days.
- ❖ 1959: The World Health Organization established a cardiovascular disease program.
- ❖ 1960: High blood pressure, one of the risk factors for stroke, was determined to be treatable. A coronary care unit (CCU) was established in Bethany, Kansas. Cigarette smoking was found to be a major risk factor for heart disease. Additionally, in that same year, Albert Starr and Miles Lowell Edwards replaced a heart valve using the Starr-Edwards mechanical valve.
- ❖ 1961: In the United States, it was determined that high blood pressure, cholesterol, and electrocardiogram abnormalities increased the risk of heart disease. During that same year, J. R. Jude restarted the human heart using external cardiac massage. Also, Bernard Lown and Barough Berkowitz used external paddles to perform direct-current defibrillation.
- ❖ 1964: In the United States, Charles Theodore Dotter led a team that performed an angioplasty to widen a narrowed artery.
- ❖ 1965: In the United States, Dr. Adrian Kantrowitz and Dr. Michael DeBakey mechanically implanted devices to aid a diseased heart.
- ❖ 1967: Dr. Christiaan Barnard of South Africa performed the first ever transplant of an entire heart.

Additionally, Dr. René Favaloro of the United States performed a coronary bypass graft for the saphenous vein. Furthermore, Framingham established obesity and inactivity as major risk factors for heart disease.

❖ 1969: Dr. Denton Arthur Cooley of the United States facilitated the use of the first artificial heart in the human body.

❖ 1970: In the United States, aspirin was recognized as a means of prevention for stroke and heart attack. During the same year, computerized tomography (CT) began to be used to aid in the diagnosis of stroke.

❖ 1972: The Stanford Three Community Study (later the Stanford Five-City Project) started in the United States. The project recorded a 23 percent reduction in the risk of coronary heart disease thanks to community-based interventions. In Finland, the North Karelia Project was initiated with the aim of reducing CVD among residents. As a result, the mortality rate of men (thirty-five to sixty-four years of age) recorded a 57 percent decrease between 1970 and 1992.

❖ 1974: In the United States, a research study conducted at Framingham State University linked diabetes to cardiovascular disease.

❖ 1977: Andreas Gruentzig of Switzerland performed the first successful coronary percutaneous transluminal coronary angioplasty. He inserted a catheter with a balloon tip in the coronary artery before inflating the balloon. He successfully restored blood flow by opening the blockage. That same year, the Martignacco Project of Italy used community-based interventions to reduce the risk of coronary heart disease. This project changed lifestyle-related factors, including tobacco use, dietary habits, and physical activity. Additionally in 1977, researchers at Framingham State University in the United States described the effects of LDL cholesterol, triglycerides, and HDL cholesterol on the human heart.

- ❖ 1978: Researchers at Framingham State University determined that psychological factors can seriously affect heart disease. In Australia, the North Coast Lifestyle program recorded a significant reduction in tobacco use in that same year. Similarly, in Switzerland, the National Research program performed a community trial that successfully reduced obesity, smoking, and blood pressure. During this same year, it was determined that an irregular heartbeat increased the risk of stroke.

- ❖ 1979: In South Africa, a coronary risk factor study performed a prevention trial aimed at reducing blood pressure, smoking, and other coronary heart disease risks. In Germany, Peter Rentrop used a clot-dissolving drug called intracoronary streptokinase to stop the progress of a heart attack.

- ❖ 1981: A study at Framingham State University found that filtered cigarettes carry an equal risk of CHD as unfiltered ones. In the same year, a report was published showing the relationship between heart disease and diet.

- ❖ 1982: Dr. Robert Koffer Jarvik of the United States designed a permanent artificial heart that was implanted in a sixty-one-year-old man by Willem DeVries.

- ❖ 1983: Dr. P. N. Hopkins and Dr. R. R. Williams of the United States published a list of 246 risk factors for coronary heart disease.

- ❖ 1984: Sir Richard Peto of Oxford University in the United Kingdom introduced a reliable method of assessing cardiovascular treatments with large-scale megatrials for minimization of random error.

- ❖ 1986: In France, French cardiologist Dr. Jacques Puel and German cardiologist Dr. Ulrich Sigwart implanted the first coronary stent.

- ❖ 1987: In Japan, Dr. Masahuru Okada revascularized a diseased heart by burning the heart muscle channels using a laser. During this same year, the Framingham

State University medical research team identified that high blood cholesterol was directly related to cardiac arrest deaths in young men.

- ❖ 1988: A study at Framingham State University found that high levels of HDL cholesterol reduced the risk of death. Also, ISIS2 trials showed the effectiveness of emergency heart attack treatment using fibrinolytic (clot-busting) drugs and aspirin. In the same year, Framingham State University researchers discovered an increase in the risk of heart disease due to isolated systolic hypertension. Cigarette smoking was also identified as a factor that may increase the risk of stroke.
- ❖ 1990: Randomized trials were conducted to show that the risk of stroke was lowered by reducing blood pressure. In the United Kingdom, Clinical Trial Service in Oxford conducted a meta-analysis of trials that showed that the risk of coronary disease was significantly reduced when blood pressure was lowered.
- ❖ 1991: In China, the Tianjin Cardiovascular Disease Intervention Program performed a community prevention trial that led to an increase in sales of low-sodium seasoning and the initiation of a no-smoking environment.
- ❖ 1992: In Canada, the Victoria Declaration affirmed cardiovascular disease as a preventable disease. The declaration meant that there was significant scientific knowledge to cure CVD. However, what was lacking was the knowledge, resources, and public health infrastructure needed to prevent the disease.
- ❖ 1992: The first heart-lung transplant was performed in China.
- ❖ 1994: The United Kingdom, the United States, and the Scandinavian nations recorded remarkable improvement in the survival of patients who had been treated for coronary heart disease.

- ❖ 1995: The Catalonia Declaration in Spain invested heavily in heart health; a follow-up investment was made in 1997. The declaration highlighted the benefits of investing in heart health and showcased success stories of CVD prevention programs across the globe.
- ❖ 1998: A hypertension gene was identified in men from the United States. In the same year, more advances were made showing that gene therapy helped grow new blood vessels. There was a strong confirmation that super aspirin IIb/IIIa receptor blocker drugs prevented blood clots. Better, though, was the recognition of the importance of cardiovascular disease inflammation. In Singapore, the Singapore Declaration was established to forge goodwill toward heart health in the coming millennium.
- ❖ 2000: In Canada, the Victoria Declaration on Women, Heart Disease, and Stroke was formed. The goal was to address the benefits of science and policy. It addressed the importance of tackling gender disparities and emphasized the benefits this would bring to overall health. The first World Heart Day was introduced; it has since grown to become a renowned annual global event. During the same year, the entire human genome was mapped. The World Health Organization endorsed a global strategy for noncommunicable disease prevention and control. It outlined the major goals of placing special emphasis on the monitoring, prevention, and management of noncommunicable diseases (NCD). The common NCDs with major risk factors include diabetes, respiratory diseases, cancer, and cardiovascular disease.
- ❖ 2001: In Japan, the Osaka Declaration emphasized the worldwide nature of the cardiovascular disease burden. It also highlighted the importance of addressing economic and political factors in a bid to eliminate cardiovascular diseases.

- ❖ 2002: In the United Kingdom, the Heart Protection Study showed how statins could help people with low cholesterol levels and diabetes. In the United States, Dr. Michael DeBakey's ventricular assist device won the NASA Commercial Invention of the Year award.
- ❖ In 2002, Alain Cribier implanted the first human transcatheter aortic valve replacement (TAVR) using an equine valve with a balloon-expandable frame.
- ❖ 2003: The framework convention on tobacco control by the World Health Organization was adopted at the World Health Assembly. The world health report titled "Shaping the Future" showed that cardiovascular disease was one of the three alarming threats comprising neglected global epidemics.
- ❖ 2004: In Switzerland, the World Health Assembly endorsed the World Health Organization's global strategy on physical activity, diet, and health. In Italy, the Milan Declaration on heart health was initiated, positioning technology as a pillar in serving global heart health.
- ❖ 2013: MitraClip became the FDA's first commercially approved alternative to mitral valve regurgitation surgery.
- ❖ 2016: The FDA approved the first pacemaker that did not require the use of wired leads to provide an electrical connection between the pulse-generating device and the heart.

Chapter 2

Mandate in Change

2.1 Overview

The strategies being adopted to reduce the rate of cardiovascular disease are not currently sufficient. Research shows that in the coming twenty years, heart disease might increase by 10 percent around the world, clearly indicating the need for new and innovative treatments.

Unless something is done fast, the rate of early death due to cardiovascular disease may increase by as much as eight million people a year in the coming years. The United Nations has plans to reduce the number of early deaths by 25 percent by 2025. The UN initiative is aimed at reducing the prevalence of CVD risk factors like tobacco use, obesity, high blood pressure, and diabetes.

Global researchers are optimistic that the plan will have desirable results. However, if nations do not rise to the task, then achievements will fall far short of goals set by the UN. While much has been done in the global fight against CVD, many gaps in prevention and treatment remain to be bridged. The hard truth is that we are not doing enough to fight the epidemic of CVD. Our current technology is insufficient to prevent and treat heart disease, though it is a promising and new advances can be built upon existing technology.

The mortality from and incidences of cardiovascular disease are declining, but the number of people disabled or affected by CVD shows no signs of decline; rather the opposite is true. For instance, the number of deaths from stroke has increased by 41 percent, stroke-related incidents have increased by 66 percent, and the prevalence of stroke has increased by 84 percent globally.

2.2 Technology and Cardiovascular Disease

The fight against cardiovascular disease includes the use of innovative technology and much knowledge derived from scientific research. Although these technologies are yielding considerable success in the reduction of acute cardiovascular mortality, cardiovascular disease has not gone away.

On the contrary, CVD accounts for 31 percent (or 17 million) of the total number of deaths worldwide. In comparison, AIDS is responsible for the deaths of three million people globally each year. Despite the enormous amount of money, resources, and research that have been used to develop and implement these new technologies, the results are not trickling down with a similar magnitude and too many people continue to die from these largely preventable and treatable diseases.

This should serve as a wake-up call. Action must be taken to fight this global health crisis. While other fields of the health-care sector continue riding high on new inventions, researchers in the CVD arena seem to fight in vain or gain a fraction of the desired result. In the meantime, people around the world continue to die at an alarming rate.

These researchers are still struggling with the burning question of which technological development needs a stimulus to deliver a monumental improvement. The most important improvements in the field of CVDs are recorded in perfect folds.

Because CVD is such a large and complex set of interconnected issues, risk factors, and diseases, it is difficult for researchers to know where best to focus their attention. No two patients with CVD will have identical risk factors, symptoms, and diagnoses so a one-size-fits-all treatment plan is impossible, making CVD is particularly difficult problem to address with technology.

2.2.1 Imaging and Processing Technology

However, the technology of heart imaging and processing is progressing in the right direction. Technology has made it very easy to visualize the heart in detail and observe its morphology and the vessels' functions. These most commonly used imaging technologies are:

- ❖ magnetic resonance imaging (MRI)
- ❖ computed tomography (CT)
- ❖ single photon emission tomography (SPECT)
- ❖ electron beam tomography (EBT)
- ❖ positron emission tomography (PET)
- ❖ intravascular ultrasound (IVUS)

Other vital molecular imaging technologies are conducted at the organ and cellular levels but while the technological techniques are still progressing and positive developments are highly anticipated, our focus will be on the use of these techniques in clinical problem diagnostics.

Noninvasive techniques in particular are showing great promise. However, considering the overwhelming preponderance of CVD, these developments are not occurring at a quick enough pace. The techniques currently in use lead to better screening for risk factors, which will be useful in identifying individuals who are at greater risk for developing CVD. In turn, this will prevent CVD-caused deaths.

Shifting away from a diagnostic approach and toward more preventative measures is key to making the biggest difference. Such preventative measures include:

- ❖ detecting atherosclerosis with an eye towards unstable plaque in coronary vessels, the iliac artery, and the carotid artery;
- ❖ providing insight into microcirculation; and
- ❖ visualizing apoptosis of cardiomyocytes.

We can extend the technological techniques to clinical problems for the prevention of CVD by a good margin. The desired destination of dramatically reducing CVD deaths is clear but the road to getting there is bumpy. Several factors must be considered and addressed including:

- ❖ Application-oriented research is needed. The new imaging techniques require a detailed validation of the practical application.
- ❖ A multidisciplinary approach by all parties is ideal, including preclinical and clinical areas of expertise.
- ❖ Great strides must be made in the development of radiopharmaceuticals for labeling and establishing biomarkers applied in molecular nuclear cardiology.

2.2.2 Digital Technology Is Not Delivering What We Need

Let's face it: the most important way to achieve commendable results in the area of cardiovascular disease prevention and treatment is digital technology. But do we have anything to show for the inputs that have been made in this area?

The answer is both yes and no in equal proportions. On a positive note, most cardiovascular diseases *are* preventable, and there is no denying that commendable steps have been made in the use of digital technologies to prevent cardiovascular disease.

Technology has changed the way stakeholders approach the prevention of this epidemic and has played a pivotal role in successes to that end. On the other hand, we have stalled in one way or another because stakeholders are working at cross purposes and have thus far failed to form a united front to work together to combat these diseases. As a result, digital technology has not been as successful as desired. Why has technology stalled?

2.2.2.1 Penetration

It is undeniable that digital technology has penetrated the healthcare market. But we cannot rest on our laurels because the lines between patients and consumers are blurring and we must reach all sectors of the field to truly be successful.

Lifestyle modification is the core of cardiovascular disease prevention. Physical inactivity, cigarette smoking, diet, and obesity are major CVD risks and addressing and mitigating those risks is the purview of much of the new technology currently on the market.

Technology is a part of increasing patient engagement and is at the center of quality patient care. Many health-care stakeholders and technology companies believe that we can achieve success through the use of sophisticated technologies. However, across the globe, the simpler, less complex technologies have been successful on a greater scale.

The traditional health-care market is not easy for sophisticated technology to penetrate and as a result, the focus must change to simpler tools for consumers like digital tracking devices such as smart watches, Fitbits, etc. These simple tools increase patient engagement, which gives patients autonomy over their own health and these devices also help to address major risk factors for CVD.

2.2.2.2 Handling Patients' Health Data

How do we collect data pertaining to cardiovascular disease? There is a big problem in the way we currently collect and handle the data for patients with cardiovascular disease in that such data is normally only collected after a patient has been hospitalized or treated for CVD or a related symptom. By collecting data retroactively, we are not helping to prevent cardiovascular disease.

Instead of waiting until there's a problem to solve, it is time to develop digital technologies that allow for a real-time analysis of patient data. The use of electronic health records is a positive first step, but there is much more that still needs to be done.

On the positive note, cardiovascular disease databases are being used in the field and in clinical trials. However, data resources should be available for patients falling outside of clinical trials. Such resources lead to the development of evidence-based medicine guidelines, quality assurance, and a resourceful point of reference for research.

Until we have registries with robust attributes (customizable analytics and interoperability) in place, results will remain elusive.

Google Play and Apple's App Store have several apps pertaining to CVD available. There are also other smartphone-based technologies that are being used in clinical trials aimed at managing risk factors and promoting healthy behavioral changes. Results are inconclusive at present. However, the American Heart Association states that the absence of evidence should not be used as proof that mobile health applications are ineffective at preventing CVD.

We must focus on producing much-needed evidence on the effectiveness of the new technologies. We must rise to the challenge and define the best methods of adopting technologies that lead to better comprehensive patient care. In the United States and in other countries across the globe, there are grants and initiatives underway aimed at bridging the gaps in digital health science.

2.2.2.3 Redefining Points of Care

Digital technology plays an important role in transforming a patient's home into a clinic or hospital. The approach to health technology should be a holistic one, not aimed solely at cardiovascular disease prevention, but rather determined to address emotional health and social connectivity through the use of technology.

Using technology in daily activities and at home will ultimately have an impact on the management and prevention of cardiovascular diseases. Currently, health technology has not redefined the patient's home as an important point of care. Patients do not consider their home in the same way they do a doctor's office of a hospital, leading to a disconnect in care. This also leads to patients not taking responsibility for their own health. And while technology has made inroads into this area insofar as wearable devices allow patients to track a number of factors from anywhere at any time, total buy in has yet to occur. Cardiovascular diseases are still on the rise despite the input and effort that has been made. In this case, the resources exist, but have not been leveraged for their full benefit.

2.2.2.4 Wide Inequalities of Smart Phones

There is concern regarding the use of technology in cardiovascular disease prevention around the widening gap between individuals who can afford mobile devices and those who cannot. Smart phones, while increasingly less expensive, are still out of reach of many people in developing and third world countries.

In developing countries, smart phone ownership is 37 percent (2015). Although this is a remarkable rise from the 2013 data (21 percent), the majority of the population in developing countries is still without access to a smart phone, making technological cardiovascular disease prevention through this method unhelpful to many, many people.

2.2.3 Major Gaps in Prevention of CVD

The reason cardiovascular disease prevention strategies are not effective is due to a number of factors discussed below.

2.2.3.1 Lack of Awareness

There is a great deal of evidence that modifying behavior is successful in treating CVD. However, the level of awareness regarding cardiovascular diseases and its risk factors remains worryingly love among the general public who lack the practical   practical knowledge about how to manage and prevent cardiovascular diseases. As a result, behavior modification has been suboptimal, which leaves room for improvement.

What is the remedy? Public awareness is at the core of the prevention of cardiovascular disease. Doctors, medical professionals, and the general public must be on the same page when it comes to their stated goal. Patients must be made aware that their role in the prevention of cardiovascular diseases is the most important. They should:

- ❖ avoid tobacco;
- ❖ eat healthier diets;
- ❖ engage in physical activity;
- ❖ manage their weight;
- ❖ know their numbers; and
- ❖ conduct personal research to increase awareness.

2.2.3.2 Are We Using Wide Population Strategies Effectively?

In 2008, it was argued that one of the greatest dangers of using the high-risk approach is its negative impact on cardiovascular disease prevention. This approach has misled planners and professionals into thinking they can accomplish the task of CVD prevention on their own.

This unreasonable focus on high-risk prevention approaches and the failure to use population-wide prevention strategies are the major reasons for inefficiency in cardiovascular disease prevention. To achieve the desired results, all stakeholders should understand their roles in the prevention of cardiovascular diseases.

2.2.3.3 False Low-Risk Assurance

Are we targeting the right group of individuals? Currently, the majority of primary prevention strategies focus on individuals with moderate to high cardiovascular disease risk. This is disadvantageous for prevention as people labeled as being low-risk are not motivated to adopt healthy behaviors. They are falsely reassured and feel comfortable that their situation is nonthreatening. As a result, many of them continue in their current lifestyles without making preventative changes and eventually, they find themselves in the high risk group. It is a classic example of waiting for a problem to develop before addressing the root cause.

According to the American Heart Association, up to 80 percent of strokes occur in low absolute risk individuals. One editorial in the *International Journal of Epidemiology* recorded a fundamental failure in the prevention strategies for these individuals who were largely ignored by the medical community prior to their strokes.

The editorial showed that prevention strategies aimed at high-risk individuals are unable to prevent cardiovascular diseases in those presenting as low-risk. Essentially, a low-risk assurance neglects the majority of the population.

Categorizing individuals into low, medium, or high risk is disastrous and does virtually nothing to prevent cardiovascular disease. It leaves a substantial part of the population out of preventive interventions.

2.2.3.4 Blood Pressure Management

The current guidelines for the absolute risk assessment of cardiovascular disease are based on the overall risk of CVD. Therefore, individuals with blood pressures higher than 140/90 mmHg may not receive antihypertensive medication because their cardiovascular disease absolute risk falls below 15 percent.

Blood pressure is an important factor in cardiovascular diseases and it is also largely modifiable. Therefore, when this level of absolute risk is neglected, there is no way our prevention strategies will have a reasonable success rate.

2.2.3.5 Ineffective Screening

Some risk factors are often missed during the screening for cardiovascular disease. This is largely due to the inapplicable behavioral risk factors in the algorithms used in CVD prevention strategies. These risk factors include the following:

- sedentary lifestyle
- chronic stress
- poor diet
- being overweight (obesity)
- excessive alcohol intake

2.2.3.6 Poor Specificity of Cardiovascular Disease Prediction Algorithms

Cardiovascular disease prediction algorithms are the only thing the health care sector currently relies on for CVD prevention. And although these predictions deliver crucial insights into the prevention and management of CVD, they are obtained primarily from studies based on the Caucasian population of the United States and are therefore inaccurate for the global population.

2.2.3.7 Cost Barrier

The cost of cardiovascular disease treatment in developing countries is increasing at an alarming rate. These elevated costs have become a barrier for low- to medium-income earners. Visiting a cardiovascular disease specialist or professional is very expensive and is expense is frequently cited as the reason why so many cases of CVD go unreported.

Screening procedures aimed at identifying high-risk individuals are expensive and are therefore less likely to be implemented in countries with poorer resources. In some cases, screening programs are not available to individuals in a socially disadvantaged population in developed countries.

2.3 Bridging the Gaps

"Mobile technology has the potential to change how health-related messages are delivered and help in the interventions that target behavior change."[3] Today, according to a report by We Are Social and Hootsuite, two-thirds of the global population uses mobile phones, affording for plenty of opportunities to utilize technology to improve research and health capabilities.

Organizations partnering together is a step in the right direction in terms of working towards technological ways to combat the spread of CVD. To that end, in June 2013, the World Health Organization, International Telecommunication Union (ITU), and the United Nations Economic and Social Council adopted the mHealth initiative in a quest to improve noncommunicable disease prevention.

According to statistical projections, there will be 6.1 billion smart phone users in the world by 2020. Therefore, delivering information about primary cardiovascular disease prevention via affordable mobile platforms will be a huge positive step in the prevention of these diseases globally.

A positive first step would be to target the use of culturally appropriate mobile platforms translated into the world's most popular languages. If we capitalize on the new mobile informational technology, we will cast a wider net to motivate and empower the general public across the globe. This would be a paradigm shift and a breath of fresh air in mass primary cardiovascular disease prevention. Capitalizing on the

---

[3] American Heart Association

preponderance of mobile phones will allow access to populations that were not previously able to find information about preventative behaviors and motivational techniques to stave off heart disease.

For cardiovascular disease prevention to be sufficiently effective, focus must be shifted from high-risk prevention to prevention on a large scale. People must be empowered and motivated regardless of their risk level. Using mobile phones to reach this population is a positive step in prevention on a global scale.

Chapter 3

Personal Devices and Apps Related to CV Health

3.1 Overview

Approximately 80 percent of cardiovascular-related deaths occur in low- and middle-income countries. By 2030, it is expected that there will be more than twenty-three million deaths annually owing to cardiovascular diseases. Coronary heart disease is one of the most severe cardiovascular diseases. It is responsible for more deaths than any other CVD. Because of this, it is extremely costly to the economy. Reducing the risk of CVD wherever possible is both a positive public health move and a good economic one. By lowering the barrier to adopting lifestyle changes such that people are able to pay attention to their health in many places including hospitals, the workplace, school, and their homes, we can lower the incidences of CVD. To meet this objective, it is important to incorporate mobile computing and communication technologies into both public health and health care. To that end, the latest advances in mobile and wireless technologies have been used in several areas of the health sector.

The main players in this area are smart phones and tablets, electronic devices which have become essential to most users in recent years. In 2012 alone, more than 1.7 billion smart phones were sold. According to a report by the International Data Corporation (IDC), there were an estimated 70.9 million shipments of tablets worldwide in 2011; that number rose to about 165.9 million in 2013. This growth indicates that within a short period of time, the use of these devices will be truly global.

The use of mobile devices and apps in the health-care industry has transformed a considerable number of practices, methods, and results in clinical practice. Smart phones are an essential device for most people and are easily available to those who can afford them. To reach the largest audience, many advanced medical software applications have been developed for different platforms. As a result, there are an array of apps available to assist health-care professionals with critical tasks such as maintenance of and access to health records, time management, clinical decision making, patient management, and medical education and training. Smartphones and other advanced apps provide great benefits for cardiovascular patients as well. By making patients an equal stakeholder in their cardiovascular health, the burden on medical professionals is lessened. However, some health-care professionals are still reluctant to adopt this technology. Though these new technologies they have a lot to offer, there is a need to establish better standards of use and valid practices for these mobile medical apps. Established standards will ensure a successful integration of advanced tools into the medical field. As a result, the quality of the available apps will increase, and safe use of those apps by health-care professionals and patients will be ensured.

3.2 What Apps Do Cardiovascular Patients Use and How Often?

Today, health-care professionals use mobile devices or tablets for tasks that used to require a computer. Smartphones and tablets allow for both communication and computing features in one place which makes it easy for an individual to access all the information he or she needs instantaneously.

Heart diseases are harmful to everyone everywhere, but they can be treated and managed. Most cardiovascular diseases result from various lifestyle factors, so a shift to healthier choices can have a dramatic impact on one's risk factors. Early detection of the primary symptoms of cardiovascular disease can help save lives and with the new technology available today, this detection is that much easier. This section highlights apps that equip medical professionals and the general public with educational tips to monitor heart rate, blood pressure, and other risk factors for CVD.

3.3 Benefits of Mobile Devices and Apps in Health Care

Mobile devices and advanced apps provide numerous benefits, to health-care professionals. They allow for informed decision making and data management as well as improved efficiency. As a result, patients with heart disease receive better care. These specific benefits are discussed below in detail.

3.4. Accessibility

Most of the mobile devices and relevant apps on the market have made health care practices more convenient. Because the devices are portable and allow for efficient communication. Users can access information instantaneously. Mobile apps are also be a good resource especially for updates regarding guidelines, reviews, news, and medical literature. Medical students no longer need to carry heavy and cumbersome books and reading materials everywhere as they can now access all the relevant information on a mobile device. These devices are convenient and can fit easily into the pocket of a lab coat.

3.4.1 Improved Clinical Decision Making

Most of the medical apps designed for doctors and medical care providers can be accessed with a mobile device. These tools are useful in clinical decision making. Clinical officers can easily find answers to clinical questions and medical students and practicing doctors can use mobile tools to access medical notes, drug references, and disease diagnoses to aid them in clinical decision making.

Mobile devices can also help pharmacists make more informed decisions. These apps offer instant access to a variety of drug information and other relevant details. Studies show there is an increase in the quality of treatment decisions when mobile devices and apps are a part of the clinical decision-making process.

3.4.2 Improved Completeness and Accuracy

Technology, especially mobile devices and apps, has improved the accuracy of documentation in both clinics and hospitals. There is accurate patient documentation of both the causes and side effects of heart disease. These apps also increase medical safety by eliminating human error. These devices have enhanced efficient and timely communication within health clinics to reduce medical errors in critical areas.

3.4.3 Increased Productivity

According to a study by the Deloitte Center for Health Solutions conducted in 2013, most physicians believe that information technology in health, including electronic health records (EHRs), mobile apps, e-prescribing, patient support tools, and mobile technologies, can improve the productivity of a medical practice. Mobile devices provide health-care professionals with improved skills which makes for better patient documentation, easier access to patient information, and improved patterns of work. When using mobile devices to retrieve information from a database, clinical experts report improved decision making and enhanced patient care. This results in improved care management and increased access to clinical resources such as lab tests, reports, and guidelines. Clinical officers who use mobile devices with patients report that they spend less time accessing and retrieving data, thus increasing their efficiency and productivity.

3.5 Mobile Devices and Apps: Future Trends in Health Care

There are several interesting trends associated with the use of mobile devices and advanced apps in the health-care sector. According to a study by Robinson in 2014, the app revolution has helped to improve the health-care system and clinical outcomes, which better enables medical experts to fulfill the great demand for their skills. It is difficult to manage the overwhelming number of severe medical cases such as heart disease, obesity, diabetes, and other diseases. Some of the challenges associated with patient care can be solved through the use of apps that can help address these issues so long as the apps support communication between cardiologists, patients, and other resources.

Access to mobile devices is growing worldwide, meaning that new opportunities are popping up for improved disease prevention for patients. As more complex diseases continue to emerge, it is expected that more mobile device apps will be invented to provide additional benefits to clinical practice. The future seems bright, and the world of mobile apps is expected to comprise an extensive database with advanced clinical decision support system (CDSS) prompts to aid in clinical decision making. There will be other kinds of mobile apps that will continue to replace the current apps with advanced features such as intelligence-oriented algorithms. It is also important to have mobile apps that can integrate with Hospital information system skills such as patient monitoring systems and electronic medical records (EMRs).

The influence mobile devices and apps play in educating people in the health-care industry is only going to increase. Clinicians and medical students predict that mobile devices and other apps will eventually replace textbooks in the health-care industry. Health care education is expected to steadily integrate these devices into their curriculum.

Full integration, however, is not without its challenges. There are concerns about the safety and security of patient data and the effect of this new technology on the clinician-patient relationship. There is also concern about the lack of educational training regarding incorporating mobile apps into health-care systems. Further, as regards integration of technology into medical education, there are doubts about the suggested measures used to guide educators, administrators, clinicians, and researchers on the integration of apps.

Ideally, guidelines and an ideal practice standard must be met before a medical app can enter the market. This standard should limit the number of apps being developed and simultaneously ensure the quality of the product. It is also important for respective bodies in charge of mobile apps to evaluate the usefulness and utility of medical apps that claim to offer therapeutic services. The application of these tactics will leave only those mobile devices and apps that have useful information that can be helpful for health-care professionals and patients.

Chapter 4

Genetic Analysis and Genetic Modification

4.1 Overview

In the future, cardiovascular disease detection will expand to include analysis of the human genetic code. Understanding the human genetic code and modifying it will prevent disease progression, which will prevent the passing on of hereditary diseases; it may also repair the damage.

4.2 Introduction

Cardiovascular disease involves a spectrum of conditions ranging from myocardial infarction (MI) to congenital heart disease (CHD), the majority of which are heritable. Many of the conditions leading to cardiovascular disease are hereditary. The research community has invested a great deal of resources in identifying and understanding the specific DNA sequence and gene variants that influence this heritability. It is a persistent challenge to work in gene discovery to find strategies to advance from genomic localization to helpful mechanism insights. The search is far from over, and more emphasis on the impact of next-generation sequencing is required. A focus on the use of stem cells to better understand how genetic variation influences heart disease is also necessary. The completion of the Human Genome Project (HGP) in 2003 provided an unprecedented opportunity for researchers to improve human health via modern technologies. Any subsequently developed technologies should involve the entire genome and identify genetically high-risk individuals. In the past, researchers have rarely focused on medical disorders the keys to which were hidden in the genetic code. However, the tides are changing and attention is increasingly being paid to determining genetic susceptibility to diseases clinicians encounter on a daily basis. The current medical research comes on the heels of discovering genetic variants that have the potential to assist in disease identification. The variants might not be the real cause of this disease, but they could be markers to help with risk assessment and improving diagnosis.

When analyzing genetic markers, researchers consider two approaches:

- ❖ gene studies that focus on single genes
- ❖ genomic studies that examine the entire human genome

Some heart diseases are caused by defects in a single gene, which is why genetic studies for these diseases make clinical diagnosis simple. Using a patient's genotyping can help to examine mutations. On the other hand, techniques such as RT PCR (real-time reverse transcription polymerized chain reaction) can be used to assess the expression of single genes. Many major risk factors for heart disease have been identified through this method. And while genetics certainly play a role in one's predisposition for developing heart disease, the impact of lifestyle changes and industrialization should not be ignored. While diet control and physical exercise are important factors in reducing the chance of developing a form of cardiovascular disease, understanding the human genome can play a huge role in preventing and treating CVD.

4.3 Genetics and Cardiovascular Disease Development

Heart disease is a family matter. Some specific parts of your family history can show a predisposition for a genetic heart disorder. Some of these factors include:

- abnormal heart rhythm
- sudden cardiac arrest
- heart failure at a young age
- seizures or fainting

Family members often share lifestyles, behaviors, environment, and, more importantly, genes that influence the risk of heart diseases. If your family has a history of cardiovascular disease, you are at high risk for developing the disease. So how exactly do genes influence the likelihood of a cardiovascular disease?

4.3.1 The Foundation of Genetic Variation

Over the past decade, researchers have recorded progress in understanding human genomes and characterizing their natural variability. The human genome comprises over twenty thousand protein-coding genes, which represent 30 percent of the entire gene sequence. The remaining 70 percent is made up of intergenic sequences that contain vital elements that regulate gene expression. Typically, five percent of the human gene sequence is comprised of coding exons that are partially translated into protein. The remainder comprises regulatory exons and introns located upstream and downstream of this coding sequence. The most common human sequence variation comprises differences in the individual pairs called single nucleotide polymorphism (SNP). Other sequence variations consist of a varying number of long or short repetitions of a similar motif in tandem, including:

- ❖ mini- and microsatellites
- ❖ deletion or insertion of various lengths
- ❖ structural variants affecting the large chromosomal region

Most of these variations are located in the nonfunctional regions of the human genome. They are neutral and have no phenotypic impact, which is why they are called markers. However, if a sequence variation occurs within the regulatory regions, it may alter the level of gene expression or protein sequence and cause notable phenotypic effects.

Some of the defective genes are as follows:

- ❖ Apolipoprotein E (APOE) gene

The apolipoprotein E (APOE) transports lipids to the body cells and tissues. This gene has a high affinity for binding to the LDL receptor. This is a polymorphic gene with three alleles, E2, E3, and E4, encoding the three isoforms of proteins—those are E2, E3, and E4, and they have different functions. The isoform E2 is linked with low LDL levels, and E4 is responsible for higher LDL levels. A recent meta-analysis established a 40 percent high risk of CVD in isoform E4 carriers. This identified a link between the APOE gene and CVD.

❖ LDL receptor gene
When the coding of this gene is defective, the functions of the LDL receptor are reduced or abolished. This results in an increase of LDL, leading to higher risk of CVD development.

❖ Familial defective ApoB100
A defective ApoB100 gene alters the binding capacity of the LDL and its receptor. This results in increased LDL levels in the blood plasma, thereby causing premature atherosclerosis.

❖ ABCA1 gene
ABCA1 is a gene that encodes proteins that monitor and regulate the efflux of phospholipids into the apolipoprotein carrier. A defective ABCA1 gene causes increased cellular cholesterol and low levels of HDL in the plasma. The alleviation of those factors shows an increase in the risk of CVD by some folds.

❖ HPA2 Met
The mutation of this gene results in accelerated clotting of the blood. This may sometimes happen even in the coronary artery. Stress and smoking are some of the factors that intensify this process.

4.3.2 Direct Genetic Predispositions

Over the years, medical research has focused on understanding the environmental causes of cardiovascular diseases. However, multiple factors are to blame. Environmental or other factors are not single-handedly responsible for CVD. Cardiovascular disease develops as a combination of the interaction between coded genotypes, initial conditions, and the exposure to environmental factors. There is growing evidence to support the argument that there is a sizable hereditary factor for most cardiovascular diseases, which is why more research is needed into genetic predisposition.

Genetic predispositions are caused by gene mutations that affect the biological functions of the original gene, thereby increasing the risk of developing cardiovascular disease. The mutations are commonly known as polymorphisms. A number of polymorphisms and linkage markers are well-known as being directly correlated to the inception of cardiovascular disease. Additionally, scientists are locating more polymorphisms all the time. The hypertension and rehabilitation department of the University of Leuven, Belgium, compiled an article detailing the polymorphisms regarded as the key factors in the development of cardiovascular disease. In addition, the genetic difference of the renin-angiotensin system has dominated current research. It is believed that these differences are the reason cardiovascular disease develops in a human being. The renin-angiotensin system is responsible for controlling blood pressure, blood flow, and other basic cardiovascular activities.

4.3.3 Indirect Genetic Predisposition

There are other genes that indirectly increase the risk of cardiovascular disease. Some of these indirect predispositions take the form of genes that make one predisposed to unhealthy behaviors that are risk factors for cardiovascular disease. For example, researchers have been looking at a predisposing gene that influences the smoking habit. Studies have shown a correlation between tobacco consumption and genetics in that some people may find it difficult to quit, and this inability eventually makes them active smokers. Because smoking and tobacco use are risk factors associated with CVD, this constitutes and indirect genetic predisposition.

4.4 Genetics and Prevention of Cardiovascular Disease

Again, some of the most common risk factors for cardiovascular disease are:

- high blood pressure
- obesity
- physical inactivity
- tobacco smoking

The primary strategies for preventing the development of cardiovascular disease have focused on the modification of these risk factors. Most of the population-based prevention strategies have focused on the utilization of primary prevention methods as a way of encouraging certain behaviors. A majority of these public campaigns and legislation methods encourage weight loss, physical activity, and stopping smoking. In developing countries where these strategies have been implemented, the results have been commendable. Additionally, these strategies have proven to be very inexpensive since they focus on the lifestyles and environmental factors of the regions and not on costly medical care. Although the methods are promising, they are also limited for a variety of reasons: They allocate precious resources to all individuals instead of putting an emphasis on those with an increased risk of cardiovascular disease. Alternative prevention strategies include utilizing individual clinical assessments, population screening, and aggressive therapy. These methods are geared toward controlling high lipids, diabetes, and blood pressure. And while the alternative methods are effective, their application is limited to the developed countries; they are often poorly applied in developing countries because they are expensive. As a result, developing countries cast a wider net with their strategies, which allows for fewer resources for high risk individuals.

The future of CVD prevention relies on new inventions. An acknowledgment of the genetic component and the correlation between the environment and genes are both crucial for developing new prevention strategies. Such interventions will bring about comprehensive risk assessment and help in optimizing population-based preventive methods.

4.4.1 Genetic Testing

Each individual's level of risk is different. Some who face a very high risk of developing cardiovascular disease can directly attribute this risk to their genetic makeup, regardless of their lifestyle and environmental factors. This genetic risk can be monogenic (involving one gene), such as glucocorticoid suppressible hypertension and familial hypercholesterolemia. Alternately, cardiovascular disease can be the result of multiple gene variations either by selection or chance. The degree of this variation varies between individuals to geo-ethnic groups. Additionally, the interaction between the environment and gene variants leads to varying results that make it difficult to predict the expression of cardiovascular disease in individuals with polygenic variants. Although medical research has established various genetic tests for high-risk individuals, the level of uncertainty is high. There are still too many unknowns because many susceptible gene-environment interactions have not been identified.

Due to its cost, it is likely that genetic testing will not be fully implemented globally for many, many years. This calls for a new understanding of the impact of genes and gene-environment interaction which can be beneficial as an argument to develop tests that can be utilized globally. Researchers can conduct constructive studies on ways to create improved genetic tests that will accurately predict inequity and effectiveness of antihypertensive medications which are frequently prescribed.

4.4.2 Population Screening

Currently, blood tests combined with the most common environmental factors provide the best prediction of cardiovascular disease. However, future genetic testing should be able to provide data that cannot be obtained via the risk factors alone. When that data is combined with the available screening strategies, the predictive power will be boosted and prevention strategies will be that much more effective. An effective population genetic screening strategy is capable of predicting the genetic characteristics unique to a specific population which can then be used to determine appropriate strategies for cardiovascular disease prevention and treatment. If done right, population genetics is capable of identifying the differences in environmental susceptibilities and genetics between populations that contribute to the disparity in cardiovascular disease prevalence. The industry has recorded major strides, but at this stage, population-wide genetic screening is not practical because of the high uncertainty of genetic testing. Given the extremely slow pace of research in the industry, this does not seem likely to change any time soon. Many countries lack sufficient funds to implement genetic testing and the research is not being done. However, the time will come when genetic screening will be an accurate prediction of the risk factors for CVD and the costs for such testing will not be prohibitive. Population screening is a precious investment for the prevention of cardiovascular disease. Making such investments will constitute a giant step forward toward a world where CVD can be prevented effectively.

4.5 Use of Genetics in the Treatment of Cardiovascular Disease

Despite all the advances that have been made, cardiovascular disease is still a major cause of mortality and morbidity worldwide. Preventing and treating this disease is a long-term fight. As previously noted, CVD is particularly difficult to treat because patients respond differently to similar methods of treatment. For instance, even with the appropriate therapy to achieve target blood pressure, the majority of hypertension patients are prone to acute MI or stroke. Additionally, not all patients react well to behavior modification. Scientific studies claim that genetic variation is the reason patients respond differently to treatments. However, the study of the human genome has presented promising options that offer effective alternatives for the treatment of this disease. For over fifty years, inheritance has been recognized as the major reason for the varying drug responses in patients, which has led to the birth of pharmacogenetics.

4.5.1 Pharmacogenetics and Pharmacogenomics in CVD Treatment

Because of the difficulty in treating cardiovascular disease, it is necessary to develop more advanced approaches for treating individual genotypes. The most recent evidence shows that combining genomic and genetic factors with environmental factors may lead to an important breakthrough. We know that genetics play a role in the way patients respond to drugs. For this reason, genetics can be used as a key factor in determining how drugs are administered. Pharmacogenetics involves the study of genetic variants that influence one's response to drugs. It includes the study of individual variations at risk for unexpected side effects of drugs and the primary domain of medication action. The study is very important in identifying genetic variants that affect the function and structure of proteins that alter the effects of drugs via metabolism, drug handling, and clearance. Pharmacogenetics can help optimize therapy and reduce toxicity via genetically guided and individualized therapy. Using this method in the treatment of cardiovascular disease can be very beneficial when making drugs that are tailored for a specific individual and that takes into account his or her ability to absorb and metabolize the drugs. This can aid in the manufacture of drugs tailored to an individual's genetic profile.

Additionally, pharmacogenomics is important for improving the care of cardiovascular disease patients by identifying individuals at high risk for toxicity. Fortunately, serious cardiovascular medication toxicities are rare because most drugs are safe. However, for those medications with serious toxicities, pharmacogenomics will help to identify risk, thereby preventing potential fatalities. Pharmacogenomics is extremely promising thanks to the potential it has to identify the source of interindividual variability affecting drug safety and efficacy. Despite its great promise, pharmacogenomics has found limited application, and is mainly used in academic referral centers. However, there is great hope that in the years to come, genetic drug responder tests will be available. These tests are predicted to help physicians individualize prescription drug therapies.

4.5.2 Gene Therapy

While pharmacogenomics and pharmacogenetics have great potential to advance current cardiovascular treatments, permanent answers have yet to be found. The current cardiovascular disease medications have the potential to alleviate symptoms and risk factors. However, there is one downside: the drugs are very powerful and have negative side effects that may prevent patients from taking medication properly. The search for a permanent solution is the main focus of modern studies in gene therapy. Upon its completion, gene therapy will involve a onetime treatment involving the introduction of a modified or normal gene sequence into a patient's genetic code to treat cardiovascular conditions.

Studies have shown that the majority of cardiovascular disease conditions are amenable to gene therapy protocols. Major experimental strides have been made, especially in the treatment of late vein graft failure, ischemia, hypertension, thrombosis, and atherosclerosis.

Chapter 5

Telemedicine

5.1 Overview

Telemedicine is when medical services are provided over a distance using technology such as with videoconferencing or the like. In rural or remote areas where many of the specialized medical services the community requires are unavailable or unreachable, telemedicine can be a viable and reliable alternative.

In the case of tele-audiology, remote tests have been found to be equivalent to those same tests done in person. Although little research has been done into tele-audiology, it is a hugely important area because of the developmental problems and the quality-of-life issues that often affect those with hearing loss. The majority of the global population does not have easy access to the hearing health services. Tele-audiology is just one example of telemedicine. This chapter will discuss the potential applications of telemedicine as well as its advantages and disadvantages.

The introduction of new technologies in health care and the advancement of telecommunications have fostered the rapid growth of telemedicine. These new information and communication technologies (ICT) allow for innumerable possibilities in the exchange of information about health and have begun to make possible new forms of assistance. These include those carried out at a distance between the health professional and the patient.

Initially, the main goal of incorporating information and communication technologies into the health sector was to make health services available to people residing in remote areas. They were also understated in order to improve the accessibility to them. Subsequently, a second evolution took place in which these technologies were transformed into instruments for improving quality of care. This made it possible to support the decision making of health professionals located remotely. Recently, these new technologies have functioned as a tool to improve efficiency in public and private health services. These tools enable sharing and coordination of resources that are separated by geography. They also allow for the redesign of health services to adjust resources to this new environment.

The prevalence of CVD calls for efficient and more advanced strategies of health-care delivery. This includes a new approach that encourages individuals to effectively manage their care without being overly reliant on consultations with costly health-care professionals.

The shift to self-management is a breath of fresh air to health care. It will boost the positive outcomes for health care and reduce costs, thereby encouraging more people to take part. The current provisions use technology to achieve this goal. Many countries envision remote monitoring, the Internet, and telephone support as the end game to providing full care to everyone.

Is it therefore good to consider telemedicine and telehealth and explore their potential for transforming health-care delivery in the fight against cardiovascular diseases. The literature on the use and effectiveness of telemedicine and telehealth is growing, and it is time to shed more light on the promise of these applications. How will telemedicine and telehealth help in the prevention and treatment of cardiovascular conditions? We need a grasp of the basics before we can explore in depth. First, we need a definition of telemedicine and telehealth.

5.1.1 Telemedicine

Telemedicine is the practice of providing health-care services using information and communication technology. It is commonly used in situations where the patients and the health-care professionals are not in the same physical location. ICTs have shown great potential for addressing the hurdles faced by developed and developing nations in providing cost-effective, accessible, and high-quality health-care services.

Telemedicine uses technology to deliver valuable information for diagnosis, prevention, treatment, research, and the evaluation of a disease or medical condition. Telemedicine is utilized to advance the health of individuals and their community.

Telemedicine helps with overcoming geographic hurdles to provide easier access to health-care services. This is hugely beneficial for underserved communities in the rural areas, particularly in developing countries, but it can help all communities that do not have access to proper health care.

Telemedicine involves the exchange of valid medical data and information via sounds, texts, images, or other forms of data needed for the diagnosis, prevention, treatment, and follow-up care of an individual.

Pertinent to our interests are the ways telemedicine can help in the fight against cardiovascular diseases. Telecardiology, for example, is beneficial in treating CVD. Telecardiology occurs in three applications: prehospital, in-hospital, and posthospital.

- In the prehospital application, telecardiology utilizes a twelve-lead electrocardiographic diagnosis for prior detection of acute MI. The information is communicated to the emergency physician before the patient arrives.
- In the hospital application, telecardiology is utilized for communication between small hospitals in underserved areas and the larger, main hospitals to improve access to echocardiography diagnostic tools.
- In the posthospital application, teleconsulting between specialists and general practitioners, telenursing, and

the diagnosis of arrhythmias are made easier with telecardiology.

The use of telemedicine for the diagnosis or treatment of cardiovascular conditions has been around for more than ten years. PubMed has more than five hundred examples of research and studies in telemedicine. This speaks to the efforts being made to incorporate telemedicine as part of the prevention and treatment plans for cardiovascular diseases.

Telehealth, compared to telemedicine, deals with a broader spectrum of remote health-care services. The term "telehealth" was coined in the early 1970s and refers to methods of conducting medical consultations using video communication. Since then, the meaning of the term has been broadened to cover all strategies of health-care delivery used to overcome geographic barriers.

5.2 Application of Telemedicine

Telehealth is one of the best ways of eliminating inequalities in the prevention and treatment of cardiovascular diseases. In doing so, it makes resources broadly available in a timely manner to those in rural areas. Telemedicine provides an effective platform that encourages individuals to adapt to a healthier lifestyle in order to reduce the risks of cardiovascular diseases.

Telehealth contributes across the full scope of care including:

- primary and secondary prevention
- acute care
- rehabilitation
- CVD management
- palliative care

The advent of both mobile and fixed broadband connections has made it easier to engineer effective ways of implementing telehealth for cardiovascular disease prevention and treatment. Additionally, the near-universal ownership of mobile devices has contributed to the growth of telehealth and now includes telemonitoring and behavioral applications.

5.2.1 Primary and Secondary Prevention of Cardiovascular Diseases

How does telemedicine aid prevention of cardiovascular diseases? Telemedicine is vital in supporting early diagnosis by detecting chest pain in primary cardiovascular care.

In one study, two hundred general practitioners were equipped with a mobile electrocardiograph and a telephone line to transmit twelve-lead electrocardiograms. A cardiologist was available twenty-four hours a day for teleconsultation. The telecardiology service recorded 97.4 percent sensitivity, 86.9 percent diagnostic accuracy, and 89.5 percent specificity for chest pain assessment, meaning that even without a cardiologist personally conducting exams, the results of the telemedicine were very accurate.

This demonstrates the potential for telecardiology to be a helpful tool for home management of developing atrial fibrillation. In particular, telemedicine is useful in conditions like asymptomatic atrial fibrillation. The flexibility of telemedicine is vital for frail, elderly patients in underserved populations. It will help reduce the number of patients admitted to hospitals for suspected life-threatening cardiac arrests as preliminary symptoms can be detected earlier and at a geographic distance.

5.2.2 Acute Care

5.2.2.1 Acute Coronary Syndrome

One of its most valued uses of telemedicine is the ability to transmit patients' ECGs to cardiac centers where physicians and specialists can interpret them and facilitate quick access to care. ECGs are sent by rural hospital staff, paramedics, rural general practitioners, and other emergency services. Prehospital electrocardiograms have been used for over a decade. A systematic review conducted in 2012 compared five studies using telemedicine intervention. The study found that telemedicine was a positive influence in rural areas. A meta-analysis of three of these studies demonstrated a decrease in in-hospital mortality.

Effective telemedicine interventions will lead to improved results in underserved areas. It will provide effective channels through which cardiologists can offer better advice and treatment for rural health services. However, the transmission of ECGs is just one of the core aspects of rural cardiology service. Other aspects, such as the use of helicopters to transport CVD patients, should be considered as well. Additionally, a proper combination of point-of-care testing, ECG transmission, and implementation of proper protocols for effective transfer and treatment must be established.

5.2.2.2 Acute Stroke

Another major area in which telemedicine delivers positive results is with acute stroke. With this CVD condition, there is a small window of opportunity for effective treatment. Telemedicine offers a better chance by combining clinical assessment and brain imaging with the input of neurologists – even if they are geographically distant - to deliver proper treatment. In particular, telestroke services have been implemented across the globe in order to offer patients in remote and rural areas access to neurological and radiological expertise. The horizontal-network model allows hospitals of a similar caliber to support one another. Additionally, the out-of-hours on-call model has been applied effectively in various urban centers.

It has been determined that patients' outcomes, efficacy, and safety are the same when thrombolysis is delivered in person and via telehealth. Studies have also recorded an increase in the rates of thrombolysis in rural areas, meaning that access to telemedicine is even more important.

5.2.2.3 Heart Failure

Telemonitoring, which uses equipment with remote data transfer capabilities is a unique procedure that makes it easy to obtain vital statistics for patients. These include:

- blood pressure
- blood sugar
- heart rate
- peripheral oxygen saturation
- electrocardiogram

This data is transmitted through Bluetooth, Wi-Fi (wireless fiber network access), or telephones to private health companies or hospital-based remote health-care centers.

To date, five modes of noninvasive transmission are used:

- video consultation;
- automated device-based telemonitoring;
- interactive voice response; and
- web-based telemonitoring.

Each of these transmission types allow health-care providers to remotely screen data and closely monitor patients without office visits. Trained specialists or nurses can alert their patients when an abnormal parameter is detected during a screening. Additionally, physicians are informed when to change medications or adjust management strategies before the patient's clinical condition deteriorates.

Studies have shown that these methods can successfully decrease the rate of mortality from heart failure as well as reduce hospital admission or readmission rates. Additionally, numerous meta-analyses and systemic reviews have found that telemonitoring interventions can substantially eliminate the heart failure admission rate and mortality rate and can lower the cost for improved quality of life.

5.2.2.4 Telemedicine in Arrhythmias

Arrhythmia is the leading cause of stroke, sudden cardiac arrest, and syncope. It is a life-threatening condition that is usually under-detected but has the potential to cause serious morbidity.

Telemedicine provides a platform for highly individualized medical management of arrhythmia.

Cardiac implantable devices can support remote monitoring, allowing for the monitoring and evaluation of multiple aspects of cardiovascular risk and physiology in patients. The following can be monitored with such devices:

- device function
- cardiac rhythm
- cardiac risk
- blood pressure valve
- level of compensation for congestive heart failure
- device status
- response to therapies

All of these parameters can be assessed using advanced electronic detection and reporting systems. Remote monitoring and assessment reduces visits to emergency departments.

Compared to the standard follow-ups conducted during an office visit, telemedicine's remote monitoring feature has improved the quality of health care by increasing efficiency for care providers. Home monitoring is a feasible practice that allows for early diagnosis of both technical (device-related) and medical events.

The use of a continuous wearable ECG monitor for up to twenty-four hours has been clinically validated. Such a device can be used for remote transmission of body temperatures, heart rate, respiratory rate, ECG rhythm, and variability, which may increase the rate of diagnosis of arrhythmia and improve treatment strategies. If a patient can be monitored remotely and constantly, early warning signs can be detected and treatment options can be implemented with fewer delays, thereby leading to better outcomes.

5.2.3 Rehabilitation

5.2.3.1 Cardiac Rehabilitation

When myocardial infarction is detected, it is standard practice for patients to participate in a cardiac rehabilitation program. This is typically a six-week program that involves dietary modification, graded exercise, and tobacco cessation. Patients who follow this program have shown improved risk factors and a reduction in the rate of further infarctions.

Unfortunately, the majority of MI patients do not participate in such a program, and most of those who do begin a rehabilitation program fail to complete the process. There are many reasons for this including distance, cost, and lack of information about the necessity of the program. Statistics show that patients from rural areas are disproportionately affected by these barriers.

Alternative strategies to cardiac rehabilitation programs are necessary; this is where telemedicine comes in. A systematic review of the alternative methods of cardiac rehabilitation process shows that telehealth, home-based, and Internet-based cardiac rehabilitation procedures are just as effective as in-person rehabilitation in hospitals.

Studies show that the use of mobile interventions that link patients to local resources is cost-effective and reduces inequalities in care. Unfortunately, there is scant evidence to support the use of telehealth interventions in reducing inequalities at the population level.

5.2.4 Cardiac Surgery

Assessment before the operation and postoperative follow-ups for cardiac surgery utilize telemedicine, particularly in increasing access to pediatric cardiology services.

According to one systematic review of four clinical trials involving an economic analysis of care, a reduction in travel distance reduces the cost of treatment. But despite the cost-effectiveness, the results were mixed. Additionally, an Australian descriptive study for telehealth in pediatric cardiology showed that telemedicine improves individuals' symptoms and the functional status.

5.3 Challenges

Telemedicine has helped smaller hospitals in rural areas improve the quality of their services. These hospitals have recorded a higher rate of telemedicine implementation than those in metropolitan areas because rural facilities have a more difficult time coping with travel times, population constraints, and lack of trained specialists. If applied appropriately, telemedicine can positively influence the entire care industry in both rural and urban areas.

Despite the promise, telemedicine faces multiple barriers that threaten to hamper its potential. Challenges include:

- Financial issues. Medicare does not reimburse many of the associated costs. What reimbursement does exist is mainly limited to certain institutions, rural areas, and certain CPT (current procedural terminology) codes. This is because there is a fear that telehealth will make it easy for health-care service providers to overutilize it, thereby driving up the costs and abusing the health-care system.

- Legal issues. Team members or health-care systems are required to transmit physiological information about patients. Thus far, there is no established protocol for determining responsibility among institutes, physicians, and patients so that sensitive medical information is protected.

- Technical issues. Telemedicine places a great technical demand placed on diagnosis accuracy, data transmission assurance, and timely feedback, either in twenty-four-hour or continuous daytime monitoring. This can be difficult to maintain.

The future of telemedicine depends on how regulators, providers, and payers address these challenges. Even with these challenges, telemedicine carries great promise for better and more efficient health-care services.

Chapter 6

The Positive Psychology Path to a Cure

6.1 Overview

Positive psychology is a discipline founded on the science that emotional health is more than the absence of disease. It is dedicated to the scientific study of what makes people or communities thrive and what makes those within these communities live a good life. Initially, psychology focused on psychopathology and emotional pain and finding ways to avoid and overcome pain. Psychologists ignored studying people who feel full, happy, and fulfilled. Positive psychology focuses on the study of these positive qualities and attempts to uncover methods for how to develop them because they help individuals live more fulfilling lives. Positive psychology does not ignore problems or psychological disorders. Rather, it complements traditional psychology and studies it from a different perspective. A person may not be depressed or have any emotional problems or psychological distress, but he or she can still struggle to find happiness.

Poor psychological health, including anxiety and depression, may result in severe cardiac outcomes. However, there is a great deal of evidence to suggest that concepts of positive psychology such as happiness, gratitude, and optimism are linked to better health habits. Positive psychology also has a superior cardiac diagnosis for people both with and without cardiovascular disease. Recent studies on positive psychology aimed at promoting well-being have shown positive results for patients with heart disease as well. Further data is necessary in order to identify the accuracy of these findings and its applicability to public health.

Depression disorders are common in those with cardiovascular disease; such disorders lead to poor outcomes and high costs.

The risk of a cardiovascular disease isn't constrained to those with depression and anxiety disorders but it has been associated with cardiovascular disease events related to stress, worry, anger, anxiety sensitivity, social isolation, phobic anxiety, somatic depressive symptoms, and a combination of negative affectivity. These findings indicate that standard processes associated with negative emotions may increase the risks of cardiovascular disease.

6.2 Effects of Mood, Depression, and Anxiety on Cardiovascular Health

Psychological risk factors associated with cardiovascular disease can be divided into three main types. The first includes adverse effects like depression, anxiety, anger, and distress. The second is personality patterns, specifically the type A behavior pattern and the type D personality. And the final type consists of social factors including social status and social support. Depression and anxiety are the key risk factors for cardiovascular disease recognized among both younger and older adults along with other risk factors such as sleep difficulties, obesity, substance use, or an inactive lifestyle.

The most common psychiatric diagnosis for anxiety disorders is the twelve-month prevalence rate of 17.7 percent that has a high prevalence of 30.5 percent in women and 19.2 percent in men. Several anxiety disorders develop during childhood and may persist into adulthood if not treated early. The most common among are panic disorder, social anxiety disorder, generalized anxiety disorder, and agoraphobia, though there are others.

There is no clear explanation of the link between anxiety and adverse cardiovascular events in patients with cardiovascular disease. However, recent studies show that in patients with coronary heart disease, anxiety may be responsible for mortality and cardiac arrest.

Depression and anxiety are more prevalent in patients who suffer from acute coronary syndrome (ACS). Despite how often they occur, these psychiatric symptoms may go unrecognized and can remain persistent for months or years.

Sertraline, an antidepressant group of drugs, conducted a randomized trial on ACS patients who went to the hospital with acute depression. About 94 percent had symptoms of acute depression for more than a month, 61 percent for over six months, and a significant number had experienced a major depressive episode.

Studies also show that despite the frequency of depression in this cohort, depression remains unrecognized and untreated for most patients with ACS.

Anxiety is also common among patients suffering from cardiovascular disease. High levels of anxiety are reported in 20 to 50 percent of patients with acute CV, most of whom frequently experience severe symptoms of anxiety. Studies show that anxiety may persist after cardiac events in patients who experience anxiety after acute coronary syndrome. Evidence shows that patients suffering from acute coronary syndrome have a higher chance of experiencing anxiety, with rates ranging from 16 to 42 percent.

Anxiety disorders are more prevalent in cardiac patients compared to the general population and depression symptoms often go unrecognized by clinicians. When they are recognized, follow-up with these symptoms is limited.

6.3 The Relationship among Depression, Anxiety, and Negative Cardiac Results in Patients with Cardiovascular Disease

People who suffer from depression without the presence of a cardiac disease risk suffering from coronary artery disease. According to a study by Johns Hopkins that examined precursors of depression in male medical students, depression can be used to predict the development of cardiac disease. Since the study was conducted, numerous other studies have been done on both men and women to determine the link between depression and cardiac disease. Analysis from this population indicates that depression could result in a 60 percent increase in cardiac illness. Patients with depression after being diagnosed with acute coronary syndrome are more likely to develop cardiovascular events than patients who are not depressed. Also, patients with depression as a result of an acute coronary syndrome suffer from negative cardiac outcomes. For example, post–myocardial infarction depression can be linked poor health, regular cardiac events, and increased mortality as well as other demographic factors.

Similar trends can be seen with anxiety. Patients with elevated anxiety may have higher chances of developing coronary heart disease than individuals with no anxiety. Specifically, worrying is a major stress element associated with cardiac disease. Like depression, elevated anxiety as a result of myocardial infarction is accompanied by longer incidences of cardiac complications and mortality.

Although there is a significant difference among anxiety disorders, anxious people may overestimate the danger associated with their situation and may activate a fight-or-flight reaction. In this case, the adaptive response can be potentially harmful and toxic as it has been linked to incidences of anxiety, which leads to increased risk of cardiovascular disease, inflammatory disorders, and diabetes. There is also some evidence to suggest a relationship between cardiovascular disease and psychological factors including anger, hostility, and metabolic syndrome. These issues require prompt attention.

A recent survey from the Women's Ischemia Syndrome Evaluation (WISE) discovered that the majority of women with depression and high levels of anxiety were more likely to suffer from acute cardiovascular outcomes than depressed women with low levels of stress. Depression and anxiety seem to be linked to cardiovascular outcomes for patients with ischemic disease. In most cases, depression seems to be related to cardiac events in both short- and long-term incidences.

6.4 How Positive Psychology Can Improve Cardiovascular Health

There have been multiple trials in the management of depression, anxiety, and other psychological states among cardiac patients. Most of these haven't led to substantial improvements, but there has not been a great deal of focus on efforts to increase positive psychological states, especially for cardiac patients, despite the link between positive states are healthy cardiovascular results.

Research shows that negative emotional states result in poor outcomes for patients with heart disease. There is a strong association between depression and cardiac events for patients with acute cardiac issues such as congestive heart failure (CHF) or acute coronary syndrome. These symptoms have also been linked to severe cardiac events that may lead to death. Efforts to treat depression and anxiety for patients with cardiac conditions have not yielded positive outcomes.

Unlike negative states, active states such as optimism can result in healthy cardiovascular outcomes in individuals both with and without heart disease. In a study conducted by WISE comprised of more than 97,000 women, women in the upper 25% of optimism had lower incidences of coronary heart disease and cardiac mortality compared to those in the bottom 25%. For patients who have heart disease, vigor, optimism, and well-being are linked to reduced mortality and fewer treatments. A study conducted to determine the relationship between optimism and good health indicated that optimism was associated with lower mortality and strong cardiovascular results. Further studies show that a variety of positive psychological factors such as optimistic emotions lead to healthier outcomes.

6.5 How Do Positive Psychological States Affect Cardiac Outcome?

Optimistic people tend to eat healthier and smoke less than pessimists. Additionally, adults with positive beliefs seem to have increased rates of physical activity compared to those who are more negative in their outlook.

Studies show that patients who exhibit good moods before cardiac surgery have a greater chance of adhering to postsurgical medication routines, which, in turn may have a positive impact on physiology. Optimism is associated with reduced inflammation and healthy autonomic function, which are key determinants in severe cardiac events. These can be useful factors that can have a positive impact on cardiac health.

Positive psychological states are essential and can be taught. In real life – as opposed to controlled clinical trials – it appears that a huge amount of a person's happiness results from static factors such as external events and intrinsic disposition. About 40 percent of happiness is up to an individual's control, but interventions can lead to positive emotions.

Positive psychology aims to increase the intensity of positive emotional experiences. Interventions in positive psychology focus on different activities, including acts of kindness, gratitude, optimism, and the use of individuals' strengths. A recent study on positive psychology interventions comprised of over four thousand subjects indicated that positive responses could lead to a reduction in depression, an increase in happiness, and an improvement in a person's health. A small amount of medical programs include portions of positive psychological interventions, but such exercise is still rare.

There is a real opportunity to create a positivity-based treatment for patients with acute coronary syndrome and congestive heart failure. Doing so would improve overall outcomes in the most vulnerable populations. There is a great deal still to learn about the proper method and delivery of positive psychology interventions for patients. But if the intervention is feasible, accepted, and successful in improving positive emotions, such interventions can yield significant health benefits for ill patients.

Heart disease is currently the leading cause of death in the world. Cardiologists and health experts have been working to find an ideal way to improve heart health. Recently, a new field known as positive cardiovascular health has combined the study of cardiovascular health and positive psychology. This is an attempt to establish a new method for building healthy hearts across the globe. The movement provides preventive measures instead of diagnoses, conditions, and treatment of cardiovascular disease.

6.6 Keeping Heart Disease from Getting Worse

Cardiovascular disease needs immediate attention. Drug therapy is a primary treatment option for heart disease, but other new medications are also reliable options. The next section explores the latest promising modes of medication treatment for each form of cardiovascular disease. While this list is not exhaustive, these drug models are the basis for the development of potent drugs for treating cardiovascular diseases.

6.7 Treatments for Cardiovascular Disease

6.7.1 Psychotherapy

Psychotherapy can help cardiac patients improve due to their practical sessions. Psychotherapy is a holistic approach that can also be helpful in assisting patients with other delicate situations in life. Psychotherapy interventions help reduce symptoms of depression and improve an individual's quality of life. The use of interpersonal psychotherapy (IPT) rather than active control does not yield a positive result. Cognitive behavioral therapy (CBT) has shown positive results in the treatment of anxiety disorders in patients with cardiac conditions. Additionally, several other supportive psychotherapeutic interventions have been tried on patients with cardiovascular disease, and although there have been fewer studies on these interventions, they generally improve cardiac outcomes. Psychotherapy is an effective way to treat depression and anxiety, but it may have less of an impact on medical results than traditional treatments involving the prescription of antidepressants.

6.7.2 Exercises and Rehabilitation Centers

Physical exercise is also an effective method of reducing anxiety that also offers significant cardiovascular benefits. Studies show that a regular exercise plan of continuous walking or jogging for thirty minutes, three or four times a week can be useful in the treatment of depression in patients with cardiovascular disease.

Cardiac rehabilitation programs can also help to continually evaluate cardiac patients with depression. These programs also offer social support. Both interventions can be used to treat anxiety in cardiac patients. However, depressed cardiac patients are likely to fail to exercise or are less likely to attend a cardiac rehabilitation program. Anxiety can also be a contributing factor that holds some patients back from attending these programs. Patients suffering from depression and anxiety should try medication and psychotherapy before participating in exercises and cardiac rehabilitation programs.

Positive psychology can help an individual feel happier or experience a lasting effect of stability and well-being. This form of psychology is relatively independent of a person's living environment. Therefore, temperament is one of the most important predictors of how positive a person is likely to be (Seligman, 2005).

65

Chapter 7

New Technology

7.1 Overview

The fatality of cardiovascular diseases has forced researchers to search for ways of preventing and treating this medical condition. Significant advances are based on modern technology, and they have brought hope to physicians and patients suffering from CVD. This chapter will shed more light on innovative technologies for diagnosing and treating cardiovascular diseases.

7.2 Total Artificial Hearts (TAH)

A total artificial heart is a replacement for a patient's entire heart. The artificial heart is put into the body after the biological heart has been removed.

These artificial hearts are powered by electricity and compressed air. A cable is used to connect the control console to the heart; the console can be small and portable and includes batteries and can be worn on a vest or a belt. It can also be a large box with wheels that allows a patient to move more freely within a hospital.

The main advantage of the artificial heart is that a patient's immune system will not reject it because it is made of plastic and metal, not organic material. This enables the body to work *with* the artificial heart instead of attacking it as living tissue. However, artificial hearts do not work as effectively as biological hearts. Surgery to fix an artificial heart, just like any other type of surgery, can cause infection and bleeding.

A permanent artificial heart can allow a patient to live for several years while a temporary model can give a patient enough time to live until he or she can receive a transplant of a biological heart.

7.3 Left Ventricular Assist Device (LVAD)

The left ventricle is the heart chamber that pumps blood to the aorta, the artery that leads out of the heart to other body parts. In case of a heart attack or if the heart is too weak to pump blood to the body, an LVAD (left ventricle assist device), is needed. An LVAD is a mechanical pump that helps pump oxygenated blood. Unlike an artificial heart that replaces the entire heart, an LVAD helps a weak biological function more effectively. The LVAD has both external and internal components. The pump is situated next to the left ventricle with a tube that takes blood to the aorta. A cable, called a driveline, from the pump passes through the skin and connects the pump to a controller; this controller is connected to a power source, either electricity or batteries. The patient must ensure that the controller is properly connected to a power source at all times. Today's LVAD is smaller, quieter, less bulky, and more durable than earlier versions.

An LVAD can be used temporarily while a patient waits for a transplant. Alternatively, an LVAD can be a permanent solution for patients whose hearts are completely damaged and who do not require a heart transplant.

An LVAD relieves symptoms like shortness of breath and fatigue. It can also sometimes help the heart to recover by allowing it to rest. Most LVAD patients are able to return to their normal activities. However, and LVAD puts the patient at risk of internal bleeding, infection, internal failure, blood clots, stroke, device failure, kidney failure, and respiratory failure.

7.4 Robotic Surgery

Though robotic surgeries have been used since the 1980s, today they are primarily used to assist in intricate surgical tasks. Robotic surgery is performed using computer controls. The computer controls a mechanical robotic arm that has small surgical tools attached to it. Robotic surgery helps the doctor perform complex surgeries by avoiding complications. After the patient is given anesthesia, the surgeon sits at a computer console and controls the mechanical arm. The computer console gives the surgeon a magnified, 3D, high-definition view of the area to be operated on. The surgeon leads his or her team members during the operation.

7.4.1 How Is Robotic Surgery Performed?

During a robotic surgery procedure, the surgeon makes incisions and inserts the instruments into the patient's body. A camera attached to the end of the instruments ensures that the surgeon has a clear view of the surgical site. The surgeon controls the robotic arm from the computer console while guiding and supervising team members.

There are three types of robotic surgery:

- Supervisory controlled. This surgical procedure is carried out solely by the robot. The surgeon initially programs the robot with the surgical procedure, then he or she supervises the robot, which carries out the entire operation.
- Remote surgery. This is currently the leading type of robotic surgery. During remote surgery, the surgeon controls the robotic arms from a computer console.
- Shared control. In shared control, the surgeon does most of the work and the robot supervises and monitors the procedure. The robot offers stability and support to the surgeon.

Robotic surgery has several advantages:

- The surgeon can carry out a complex and delicate operation with relative ease.
- Robotic surgery can be used where other surgery methods have failed.

- There is less surgical site infection.
- There is minimal blood loss and pain.
- There is little scarring.
- Patients undergoing robotic surgery require shorter hospitalization compared to those undergoing other surgical methods.

However, like any surgical procedure, robotic surgery has its shortcomings:

- It is more expensive.
- Like any electronic device, the machines are prone to malfunctioning.
- The surgeon must undergo intense mastering of the robot to successfully operate it.
- There are risks of complications and infections.

The Food and Drug Administration (FDA) has approved the use of robotic systems for cardiology procedures and catheter ablation. Robotics enables more precise and controlled catheter manipulation than manual manipulation can provide. One benefit of this procedure is physicians are protected from the radiation field as they sit behind the console.

7.5 Stem Cell Heart Growth

The most prominent health challenges in today's world are congestive heart failure and heart attack. Researchers found evidence that a damaged muscle cell can be replaced and new blood vessels can be established to supply these new cells. This can be done using stem cells. People suffering from diseases that damage their hearts damaged now have a way to replace their damaged heart cells. Heart muscle cells may sustain damage as a result of insufficient blood supply to the heart muscle, hypertension, sudden closure of a blood vessel supplying oxygen, or a heart attack. Despite improvements in drug therapy, mechanical assistance devices, surgical procedures, and organ transplants, patients with severe heart conditions often die within five years of receiving a diagnosis. In an effort to combat this, scientists have successfully developed a human heart in a lab by using the patient's own stem cells in place of damaged cells. This is also beneficial in that it avoids the recipient's body rejecting a donor heart.

7.5.1 How Is Stem Cell Growth Done?

Stem cells taken from a patient's bone marrow are inserted into the damaged heart through a catheter. These stem cells help fix the damaged cells.

What are the risks of stem cell growth?

- The patient's immune system may reject the stem cells.
- In case of improper communication between the injected cells and the heart's electric system, dangerous heart rhythms can be produced.

7.6 Three-Dimensional (3D) Printing of Cardiac Prosthesis

The lack of options for treatment for CVD has meant that scientists developed artificial hearts some time ago. However, many of the designs currently in use are very rough, which creates difficulties when integrating them into the human body.

With this in mind, a team of researchers from the Federal Polytechnic School of Zürich (ETH Zürich) decided to take their inspiration from the biology of the human heart.

Instead of using separate parts, the Swiss team, led by Nicholas Cohrs, 3D printed an artificial heart using soft and flexible material. The heart was printed from a single piece (or monoblock) that allowed the team to design a complete internal structure with pumping mechanisms capable of detonation by silicone ventricles, which mimics the human heartbeat.

"Our goal is to develop an artificial heart that is almost the same size as the patient's and imitates a possible functioning and shape of the human heart," Cohrs said in a press release.

So far, the team has been able to test this artificial heart, which pumps a blood-like fluid with a pressure similar to that of the human heart inside the body.

However, this design remains only a proof of concept as the artificial heart is not yet ready for implantation. Thus far, the materials used were unable to last for more than half an hour or a few thousand heartbeats.

The team continues to work with new materials and make design improvements. Once perfected, this design could potentially improve the life and health of about twenty-six million people worldwide who suffer from various heart conditions.

7.7 New Pacemakers without Leads

Traditional pacemakers consist of a tiny battery-operated power source implanted under the patient's skin. Wires are used to deliver electrical impulses to the heart muscles in order to sustain a normal heartbeat.

Traditional pacemakers are reliable, but the leads are a major undoing of the entire system. In most cases, complications arising from the system involve broken leads, which cause the entire system to malfunction. Moreover, individual patients have anatomical differences that make it difficult to implant the leads.

A leadless pacemaker is a tiny, self-contained unit implanted on the inside wall of the patient's heart via a small, flexible catheter. The first version of this new pacemaker, a single-chamber pacemaker implanted in the right lower pumping chamber, is showing great promise. Future iterations will be available in the coming years.

7.8 Google Glass

Google Glass is wearable computing technology consisting of an eyeglass-like headset a user wears as one would wear glasses. It is a sophisticated minicomputer capable of taking pictures, recording videos, and transmitting data wirelessly.

This hands-free device can be utilized during medical procedures to take pictures and transmit data without contaminating the sterile surgical environment. Google Glass plays a vital role during coronary angiography, where doctors inject a unique dye into the artery to reveal blockages or narrowing; the Glass allows them to see the dye.

A small study revealed that Google Glass broadcasted sharp angiographic images to mobile devices (such as a computer or iPad). The images were accurate enough to be properly interpreted by experts who were absent during the procedure.

Further advances in technology are expected to continue to help CVD patients.

7.9 Protein Patch

If a heart muscle cell is damaged, it can lead to a fatal heart attack. Without the ability to fully regenerate, the damaged or dead cells form scar tissue which, in turn, prevents the heart from functioning optimally, potentially leading to heart failure.

A team of bioengineering and health experts have discovered a natural protein with the ability to initiate the process of normal tissue regrowth. Most of the recent studies involving pigs and mice have found that when the damaged heart muscle was patched with the natural protein, cardiac cells began to regrow. This protein helps the heart to regain near-normal function.

Scientists are hopeful that this innovation will be successful in human beings. The patch will soon be tested in human clinical trials.

7.10 Watchman

The most common type of arrhythmia is atrial fibrillation (AF). It is estimated that over 20 percent of stroke cases occur in AF patients. To reduce the risk of clot formation in the left atrial appendage (LAA), anticoagulants are widely used. However, these drugs have been shown to cause increased bleeding or fatal hemorrhage due to ulcers or cuts.

Boston Scientific has developed the Watchman LAA occlude as a means of giving patients an alternative to the anticoagulant drugs. The Watchman is a device implanted once; it is perfect for patients with conditions unrelated to the heart valve. The device is capable of closing off the left atrial appendage in the transcatheter procedure.

The procedure to implant the device takes one hour, after which the patient is admitted to the hospital for twenty-four hours. After the procedure, the patient has a forty-five-day window during which they can stop taking the anticoagulants.

The Watchman device has been in use in the European market since 2005. It was cleared for use in the United States by the FDA in 2015. It has also been approved for mainstream commercial use in seventy other nations. Currently, it is estimated that over ten thousand patients have the implant.

7.11 Less-Invasive Surgery

In 2011, a new procedure to treat heart valve disease was approved by the FDA. This innovative, less invasive surgery called transcatheter aortic valve replacement (TAVR) corrects a defective heart valve without the need for a major surgical operation.

A catheter, a small, hollow tube, is placed in the femoral artery in the groin and guided into the chambers of the heart via advanced imaging techniques. Through the catheter, the collapsed tissue valve is positioned and guided directly into the defective aortic valve. When the valve is placed correctly, a balloon is inflated to deploy the valve. This method eliminates the need for open-chest surgery.

The TAVR device has been approved for heart valve patients who need replacement aortic valves but are at high risk from standard open-heart surgery. The procedure is a significant advancement for older patients or those who cannot withstand the open-chest procedure.

In the United States, most of the patients currently undergoing the TAVR procedure have kidney or lung diseases and are therefore less likely to withstand the standard aortic valve replacement. The TAVR procedure is moving toward mainstream global use. Currently, the TAVR procedure is utilized by over 350 hospitals in the United States.

With these and other advancements on the horizon, cardiac patients can look forward to a brighter future.

Chapter 8

The Power of Collective Knowledge

8.1 Overview

During recent years, the emergence of a new type of patient, "the empowered patient" has changed the health sector. This type of user accounts for about 21.5 percent of the total number of patients in the United States. Empowered patients have arisen in parallel to the establishment of new technologies and media.

This change in the technological paradigm and the emergence of a new class of patients can be seen in the amount of health research carried out by patients rather than doctors and medical professionals. About 60 percent of patients use tools like the Internet to look up topics related to their health, and 51 percent consult these tools for symptoms when they are not well. Empowered patients use tools and devices to actively monitor their pathologies.

8.2 The Empowered Patient

Empowered patients puts the patient at the center of health services because he or she will advocate for his or her care and not rely solely on the opinion of medical professionals. Until recently, the idea that a patient participated in medical decisions affecting him or her was unheard of. Today, many patients realize that being well informed and taking the reins in the situation related to their health is vital. But there is a fine line between being empowered and being misinformed. There is so much information available to us at any given moment that it can be difficult to determine what is accurate. What does empowerment in health look like?

8.2.1 Empowerment of the Patient: What Is It?

An empowered patient meets most of the following requirements:

- Understands health conditions and the effects of disease on the body.
- Feels capable of participating in decision making in conjunction with health professionals.
- Is able to make informed decisions about his or her own medical treatment.
- Understands the need to make the necessary changes in lifestyle to effectively manage illness.
- Can ask informed questions of health-care professionals.
- Takes responsibility for his or her health and actively seeks care only when necessary.
- Actively seeks, evaluates, and makes use of the information obtained from different sources (such as the Internet).

Empowered patients understand how to navigate the many areas in the health system, including family, doctors, health insurers, health regulators, and pharmacists better than patients who allow doctors and medical professionals to make all decisions. When he or she is unsure about where to go or what to do next, the empowered patient feels safe asking for the information he or she needs.

Paulo Freire popularized the term "empowerment." Freire considers empowerment to be both a process and an outcome. The process of empowerment occurs when the purpose of an educational intervention is to increase one's ability to think critically and act autonomously. Empowerment is the result when one achieves a greater sense of self-efficacy as a result of the process.

Policy makers and health professionals see patient empowerment as a mechanism to help patients with chronic diseases. These patients can manage their health properly and achieve better treatment outcomes than those who are not empowered.

Patient empowerment is on the political health agenda in Europe and elsewhere. Evaluations of health-care patients have become increasingly important.

8.3 The Power of Information

An empowered patient has the ability to decide, meet his or her needs, and solve problems through critical thinking and exerting control over his or her life. All of this is possible through the acquisition of knowledge. If information is power, an empowered patient *must* be an informed patient. He or she must have the proper insight to understand the disease or condition and its treatment. It is up to health professionals, therefore, to transfer knowledge and skills to patients. With the appropriate knowledge and skills, a patient can choose between his or her options and act accordingly to make health decisions in his or her own best interest.

The collaboration between patients and health care providers allows for customization of treatments, preventative measures, and an increase in awareness such that patients act in order to protect themselves. Health-care professionals must ensure that patients properly understand the information and that they know how to use it correctly. Delegating responsibility gives patients full autonomy. Such patients can be trusted to be aware of when they need to seek professional medical advice and/or treatment.. Additionally, trusting patients has been shown to have positive effects on their recovery.

8.4 The Patient and the System

Patient empowerment is based on the patient's participation both in making decisions and in self-care. It also lessens the burden on the health care system since chronic disorders consume the most resources. Patients who take an active interest in their own health are less likely to suffer from these disorders. Life habits—exercise, diet, or correct medication—

can directly influence how pathologies develop. In fact, the degree to which a patient is involved is usually a deciding factor in the overall balance of treatment.

More informed and responsible patients would improve the health care system. However, moving from theory to practice is tricky. We must start by measuring the real added value of patient empowerment. Then, we can promote a change of mentality between patients and medical professionals. It is evident that it is necessary for the patient to be an active agent agent in the health system and to ensure that he or she is willing to cooperate and share the responsibility for maintaining his or her health.

8.5 Why Patient Empowerment Is Important

What follows are ten key points explaining what it means to empower a patient or to be an empowered patient and why it is important:

1. **We are all patients.** There are still health professionals who speak of the "patient" as if that person were somehow removed from what is happening. We have all been, are, or will be patients. We must stop referring to patients in the third person and defend their rights and remember that one day, we will be patients again ourselves.
2. **Education and information.** In this book, you have been told repeatedly that information is very important for patients to have. However, receiving information alone is not enough; we must also understand it and know how to interpret that information correctly.
3. **Access.** Access means that we should not have to search for the information we need. It should be readily available to us. The ability to keep up with medical journals and the latest makes it more convenient. Our mobile phones and tablets facilitate this access, making

information available to us virtually any time and in any place.

4. **Engage.** To engaged means to make decisions that will affect us directly and to understand why it is important that we adhere (or not) to treatment.
5. **Self-management.** It is crucial to monitor our health, our chronic diseases, to promote early diagnosis or to prevent diseases. Of course, the role of the medical professional remains the same, but in managing our health, we are the ones who know when to go to the doctor, and whom to see.
6. **To be the center of the medical system.** No matter how insignificant we feel in the hospital, we are the reason the hospital exists; it is here to serve us, not vice versa.
7. **Personalized attention.** We are not all the same, and our health depends on a million unique factors.
8. **Integrated care.** Health is not isolated; it exists in a context. Global health must integrate the different medical specialties and health within the social context and take into consideration environmental and genetic factors.
9. **New technologies.** The Internet (eHealth), mobile phones and apps (mHealth), wearables, sensors and trackers, and medical devices are what make empowered patients possible.
10. **Empowerment.** The empowerment of the patient is not just a change in attitude or the use of new technology; it is a fundamental change of the entire health system. All over the world, hospitals are beginning to adapt to this reality. Empowered patients are growing in number.

8.6 The Empowered Patient Revolution Is an Opportunity for Health Professionals

Empowering patients does not mean encouraging them to seek information about their problems on the Internet or from their social circle. On the contrary, fostering empowerment in patients means helping them to avoid misinformation and encouraging healthy critical thinking at the omnipresent news from nonprofessional media or unreliable sources.

Not all patients are candidates for empowerment. Since the first initiatives in health education, it has been evident that the most efficient actions are those performed on patients with chronic health problems. Additionally, not all patients have the age, motivation, and cultural level to understand and act responsibly about their illness. This is very common in the field of neurological pathologies. Patients with acquired brain damage or neurodegenerative diseases either cannot participate or it is very complex for them to participate in decision making. For this reason, the caregiver for neurological pathology patients and the interventions in empowerment of clinical neuroscience are key. The caregiver must be one of the main factors in patient empowerment for these particular patients.

Therefore, to foster empowerment, we must start with a transmission of quality information directly between the professional and the patient (or caregiver), through well-recommended sources (on the web), or by providing information on paper. Additionally, interventions to train the patient should be sought but not imposed. The patient needs to make the decision to become empowered on his or her own. A large number of patients desire and require more information; however, some prefer to transfer that responsibility to the medical team and their wishes should be respected. Spending time and resources training someone who does not want the responsibility misses an opportunity to improve on other aspects of health. In summation, transferring quality and reliable knowledge to patients allows for synergistic management of the patient's disease, enhances his or her decision-making abilities, and increases the knowledge about his or her health, all of which should result in better clinical safety.

Are interventions to empower patients effective and efficient? The simple act of a patient asking for information on his or her pathology is a reason to propose an empowerment program. It is also true that a public health system should direct resources toward those interventions that imply a better ratio in the mix of efficiency, efficacy, and patient satisfaction.

8.7 Characteristics of the Empowered Patient

If you are in the health sector or interested in welfare, you have surely heard the concept of the "empowered patient," a term that attempts to define the changes from "health users" in the past. This is largely due to the information and communication technologies and a growing concern for the health care of millions of people around the world. However, what essential characteristics define the empowered patient?

- ❖ The empowered patient takes part of the leading role in the health field. This is a person who is no longer limited to hearing a diagnosis and trying to comply with a medical prescription. The empowered patient takes an active part throughout the entire process from the diagnosis of a disease to its cure or, at least, to the more severe symptoms.
- ❖ In this sense, the empowered patient is an informed patient. According to the latest data, health is one of the most sought-after topics on the Internet. Today, the patient who arrives at the clinic already has previous information about his or her symptoms and seeks the health professional as the qualified person who can confirm or deny the data consulted.
- ❖ The empowered patient "mobilizes." The use of smart phones, tablets, or any other electronic device that, with an Internet connection, allows us to obtain data in real time is becoming more standardized. It emphasizes here the preference, increasingly more common, of patients to monitor themselves thanks to the numerous health applications that exist in the market.

❖ The empowered patient is involved in the recovery process. This patient is concerned with how to improve treatment guidelines, consults the blogs of health professionals, and actively participates in digital communities, thus adding value by interacting with people suffering from the same disease and professionals who specialize in treating it.

❖ In an environment where the chronicity of pathologies and continuity of care are two of the great challenges facing the health system, it is more necessary than ever to work in preventive medicine and to count on each patient to adopt some life habits that will result in a decrease in episodes of ill health that end in hospitalization or a surgical process. If these eventualities occur, the patient will no longer be simply a recipient of medical and pharmacological care but must be perceived as an active agent who participates and makes decisions with his or her doctors about his or her health.

8.8 Negotiation of Treatment and Therapy

An empowered or active patient is informed, thanks to the multitude of resources at his or her disposal. There is information available at a sufficient level to provide the patient with details about his or her pathology. The health personnel must be listened to by the doctor when choosing the best therapeutic or care option. The doctor must make a pedagogical effort to explain to the patient the variety of options for treatment. The health-care professional and the informed patient will consider the various forms of treatment available and choose the most suitable option after considering the pros and cons of each. Working together, they can make the most informed and appropriate choice. This is collaborative medicine made possible with responsible patient empowerment. Patients who are involved in their own health are more likely to follow medical recommendations to obtain the best results.

Empowerment among patients is growing. For example, a patient with diabetes who must measure glucose, administer insulin, reduce his or her weight, and exercise, is more likely to be balanced and alert to symptoms typical of complications such as vision problems or cardiovascular risk. This new patient is informed, an expert in his or her pathology who speaks with other patients. He or she associates with groups of patients who share his or her needs and concerns and who receive additional help such as psychological care or physiotherapy. This expert patient is useful for all others facing a serious illness such as cancer or HIV for the first time. Faced with anxiety, such patients may be hesitant to inquire about their conditions, and the informed patient who has already been through a similar process can be a helpful and valuable resource.

8.9 New Technologies and the Empowered Patient

The technological advances that have made life easier for patients with any pathology also enable telematics monitoring of their health indicators. Telemedicine will play a very important role in the coming years, and the remote monitoring of patients with certain pathologies will increase the possibilities for home care that will be essential for educated, responsible, and informed patients who will work collaboratively with health specialists to monitor their treatments and health status.

Wearable devices are a revolution in this field and serve to further empower patients. Through wearables, it is possible to access the body temperature, blood pressure, and pulse of a patient who is hundreds of miles away. All of this information can be accessed through an application installed on a watch worn by the patient. The development of mobile applications for health control by medical professionals and health specialists will allow for the adaptation of medication designed specifically for a particular patient who may need a reduction in dosage as his or her condition improves. Devices for transdermal administration that can be ordered remotely by a physician who is constantly monitoring the patient are in development.

8.10 Patient Schools

Patients are now able to interact with each other in online forums to find relevant information about the most prevalent pathologies, which generates more questions from patients, relatives, and caregivers. These types of forums are supervised by health professionals who ensure the quality of the content. They also monitor content to make sure that the information provided is based on scientific evidence. Health professionals can also organize meetings and forums where health policy makers can answer queries from patients. These websites are an alternative offered by medical institutions and are used to counter the possible risk of obtaining medical information from websites of dubious origin and content not endorsed by medical science. A website called Commented Patient School is becoming a resource for empowered patients. Mobile applications are used to give health advice to patients, to serve as diaries of a disease, or to function as an ally to the follow-up of a pathology. Health-care administrations, scientific societies, patient associations, the pharmaceutical industry, and telematics service providers should all be included in the service of empowering more patients.

Chapter 9

Monitoring Health Status

9.1 Overview

Health is an essential part of life, and today it is recognized as a social product. Any analysis of one's health must be systematic and incorporated as a life philosophy by individuals, families, friends, communities, and countries. Everyone should feel responsible for maintaining and promoting the health of themselves and those in their community.

The analysis and monitoring of the health of various populations is carried out throughout the world in different ways. Through scientific thinking, we can identify health problems, risk factors, and vulnerabilities in the overall population.

This is a unique process that integrates not only medical sciences but also other disciplines while considering social and community participation, all in the interest of achieving a more efficient analysis. The characteristics of each region, country, and community are taken into account.

The field of epidemiology has made great contributions not only to the diagnosis of health problems, but also in assisting in decision making. Statistics has also played an important role in the interpretation of the data. that are grouped by collecting the information through several methods, techniques, and tools. These tools and techniques help health professionals and communities work more effectively to guide the strategies and actions during implementation to solve problems.

Indicators have been created for use on the local, regional, and global levels. With these indicators, it is possible to evaluate the effectiveness of the actions taken in promoting, preventing, healing and rehabilitation, comparing population groups and communities, measuring trends, and developing projects.

Future of Cardiovascular Health

In some countries with a single integrated health system, analyses of the health situation at the clinical level, with the family doctor, and at the municipal level are conducted. These analyses consider the results at both provincial and national levels to ensure that all information is articulated.

This process is complex since it requires a high preparation of human resources not only in the medical profession, but also in other fields such as social communication, research methodology, history, and local culture.

Sometimes barriers and gaps arise. For example, indicators of birth, mortality and morbidity in small populations, and other factors are used as predictive indicators. Most are linked to the disease process, while only a few are linked to positive indicators of health. On the other hand, one of the most important things to consider in today's world, with its great scientific advances, is that we must not lose sight of the social determinants of health. These determinants are essential to the analysis of any health situation contextualized in each population, community, region, or country. For a truly holistic approach, the approach must be qualitatively superior compared to the biological approach that still prevails in many spaces. The social, historical, and cultural approaches must involve community participation.

9.2 Biosensors That Enable Patients and Health

A sensor has been developed that allows us to obtain information. The biosensor is an instrument that measures biological and chemical parameters that affect living beings with a biological and physicochemical component.

A biosensor is a tool or an analytical system composed of an immobilized biological material in close contact with a transducer system. This converts the biochemical signal into a quantifiable electrical signal.

A biosensor requires several parts that are joined together. These include the biological receptor itself from which the information is obtained. In addition to elements common to living beings such as tissues, cultures of microorganisms, human body substances like DNA, cells, enzymes, and substances that form part of the blood circulation or that are found in nature or are the process of synthetic biology are collected.

The transducer or sensor provides information obtained through the biological receptor, which links the other two components to create a way to classify, quantify, and observe the information that is collected. The detector uses a technique that reveals a biological phenomenon usually hidden by thermal, magnetic, optical, electrochemical, mechanical, acoustic, and other methods.

These devices have two characteristics: sensitivity and selectivity. They unite two different types of environments to obtain the desired information; the live and the inert.

9.3 How Was It Invented?

The need for safety gave rise to the search for a way of obtaining measurements of bodily substances that was fast, reliable, and affordable. This was done so that the patient could adopt the measures necessary to face health contingencies at any time. Because of the positive results, the search for similarly useful procedures continues.

Anecdotally, the first biosensors are generally considered to be canaries that detected toxic gases in mines. In 1962, this concept emerged thanks to the work of Leland C. Clark Jr., who had worked on them since 1956. Together with Champ Lyon, he built the first sensor on the rapid and reliable detection of blood glucose levels; that sensor was commercialized in 1975.

Divis suggested using bacteria as a biological element in biosensors to measure the amount of alcohol in a sample. Prior to this, thermal transducers and enzyme thermistors were used. Later, biosensors based on fiber optics appeared and are used to determine the level of CO2 and O2. The evolution of electrochemical biosensors was reviewed by Carr, Bowers, and others.

In the 1970s, thermistor-type biosensors appeared, and around 1980, Lowe introduced the optoelectronic biosensor. In the 1970s, attempts were made to build immune sensors, and during the 1980s, Liedberg started marketing them. In 1987, a pen was built for the personal monitoring of blood glucose, which has since dislodged the traditional methods of measurement. In later years, the conductimetric and redox biosensors appeared.

In recent years, an attempt has been made to produce a miniaturized electrochemical biosensor using conventional electronic devices called field effect transistors. However, further development is still required.

Currently, a new generation of biosensors called MIPS (polymers containing printed molecular memory) is available.

9.4 Analysis in Real Time

Traditionally, to analyze any biological or clinical phenomenon, it must be detected with an element called a marker. A marker can be detected using various methods such as radiation, calorimetry, and fluorescence. This is a laboratory process that does not yield results while the study is being carried out and therefore, cannot be performed in real time.

In contrast, biosensors do not require any type of marker. They are attractive because they perform an analysis of the substance in real time. This provides not only a qualitative and quantitative analysis but allows for evaluation of the movement and speed of the reaction or kinetics of the interaction, therefore revealing the fundamental mechanisms of that interaction.

Combining the receptor layers or biological receptor with transducers has given way to a variety of biosensors, the great variety of which has been developed with various physicochemical mechanisms of transduction to translate the biological interaction into a measurable and useful signal.

9.4.1 How Are Biosensors Used?

Biosensors can be used in clinical, therapeutic, veterinary, and agricultural settings, as well as industrial processes, and pollution and environmental monitoring.

In the medical field, they may be used as support in the clinical biochemistry laboratory to determine glucose and lactic acid, for example. They monitor patients outside of medical visits and constantly update on the condition of a patient with diseases such as cancer, with substances that must be controlled, such as glucose, antigens, antibodies, and cholesterol. This monitoring improves the efficiency of patient care by replacing slow and laborious studies and facilitating effective medical decision making in a timely manner.

There are some biomarkers, such as in the veterinary, agricultural, and food fields that have been successful in controlling fertility and infectious diseases in animals. The same is true in the milk, fruit, and vegetable industries with viral and fungal diagnostics and with contamination and toxins from food, such as salmonella. There have been improvements in the production and quality of fermentation, such as that for alcohol, and in the field of pollution control.

9.4.2 Who Can Use Them?

Given the ideal properties biosensors must possess (they must be specific, discriminant, reproducible, accurate, safe, adequately sensitive, quick to respond, miniaturized, useful for small volumes of measurement, independent of temperature, cheap to produce, reliable, and requiring little maintenance), they are not universally available. However, with simple training, biosensors can be used by all types of personnel in each medical field.

An added benefit of biosensors is the fact that direct, continuous, rapid, and highly sensitive measurements can be obtained. Likewise, the advantage of portability allows for biosensors to function anywhere, whether that be in a doctor's office, at home, or virtually anywhere else.

9.4.3 Functions and Applications

Biosensors are considered the modern guardians of health and their function is to replace or complement ongoing studies. They can also conduct conventional analyses and have different characteristics to make them practical, simple, and reliable.

The application of biosensors has provided the advantageous opportunity to solve problems and to foresee repercussions in every field in which they are used. Their future potential is virtually limitless.

There is a diversity of functions and specificity of biosensors available. Patient safety, agri-food, and biomedicine have been used in the European project in the environmental field. The products in this field have been designed for the analysis of water quality in an automatic, fast, and low-cost way called WOLA (water on-line analysis, Europe).

There are many popular applications for biosensors in the field of environmental pollution or the detection of circulating blood glucose for monitoring diabetic disease. In addition, studies are being conducted on biosensors in carcinogenic detectors, drug detectors, wine evaluation, and so on.

9.5 Biosensors for Diabetics

The use of medical biosensors began with diabetes patients and their need to monitor blood glucose levels. This is the most successful and widespread biosensor in the world and has progressively improved over the years. It is a small device that recognizes an enzyme called glucose oxidase. A patient can deposit a small drop of blood on a designated strip and identify the level of glucose in his or her blood at that moment. The patient then uses those results to control his or her diet and medication accordingly.

Currently, work with biosensors implanted in type-1 diabetics (popularly called juveniles) is being done. These biosensors are involve a thin cannula connected to a portable device that constantly monitors and records glucose levels under the skin of the abdomen.

This is very useful for conveniently administering the proper doses of insulin for the patient. It can also be used to avoid the problem of overdosing and the serious consequence of hypoglycemia, which is low blood glucose caused by insulin. This device still requires clinical experience to function as an "electronic pancreas."

9.6 Other Particularities

At present, there are a variety of applications for biosensors. In the field of biomedicine, there is support for the control of metabolites, which are critical during surgical interventions in the consultation and emergency services. This can also help to prevent or curtail expenses and accelerate a diagnosis which allows for a faster start to treatment.

Additionally, there are pregnancy tests and glucose control aids for diabetics, which are available for use in the domestic area.

In the fields of industry, the military, and environmental applications, biosensors are used in food (for example, in determining the freshness of fish), cosmetics, fermentation control and quality, detection of explosives and gases that attack the nervous system, and pollution control. Biosensors are also designed to detect the remains of herbicides and prevent them from reaching food.

Biosensors are proof that a revolutionary way of preserving life and health is upon us. There is a need to adapt to a new form of disease control and early detection of contaminants, particularly in food. These can be conducted by simple, convenient, inexpensive, and rapid methods that can help an individual control his or her health.

9.7 Artificial Intelligence and the Treatment of Diseases

Techniques by imaging, information management systems, and connectivity between patients and professionals are a few of the admirable advancements in health technology. These innovations represent a monumental step forward in the areas of prevention, early detection, and the control of diseases.

However, in an aging society with the prevalence of chronicity growing at accelerated rates, a new challenge has become evident: can diseases be anticipated? In this field, artificial intelligence through big data or machine learning is positioned to become the great ally of primary prevention and health care in the coming years.

Automatic learning or machine learning identifies patterns among millions of different pieces of data (big data) and predicts behaviors through algorithms that can learn and evolve based on experience.

In the health field, the predictive analyses generated by this discipline could put us one step ahead of certain diseases and would lead to an early, precise, and decisive diagnosis in the development of some pathologies.

In the case of neuronal diseases such as Alzheimer's, in which the first symptoms can begin to occur up to ten years before the first cognitive alterations are identifiable, the possibility of anticipating the visible appearance of the disease plays a fundamental role in its development.

Currently, one of the tests most used in the early detection of Alzheimer's is called the "test of the clock," a test wherein the patient draws a clock with a certain time and has to copy another picture that has already been drawn. This practice allows professionals to observe and identify symptoms of brain deterioration that could indicate the presence of cognitive alterations.

A group of scientists led by the Laboratory for Artificial Intelligence and Computational Sciences of the Massachusetts Institute of Technology (MIT) developed a computer program capable of detecting Alzheimer's disease and obtaining a more accurate diagnosis. Compared to the earlier clock test, it uses a more objective and rigorous method of detection.

The system, based on information gathered from hundreds of previous tests, interprets data from new tests performed through a digital pen. In this way, it increases the accuracy of diagnosis. Most importantly, it helps and promotes medical decision making based on objective and comparable data.

However, once the disease is diagnosed, health systems begin the most important stage of the health continuum: personalized treatment and therapy adapted to the needs of the individual.

9.8 Artificial Intelligence for the Care and Treatment of Diseases

Chronic diseases such as diabetes, chronic obstructive pulmonary disease (COPD), heart failure, or high blood pressure need continuous monitoring and require frequent decision making.

The latest monitoring systems allow patients to improve their health status by providing them with constant updates to the most relevant indicators. Heart rate, sleep patterns, or physical exercise are some of the variables analyzed. These tools can help establish patterns of behavior based on patients' activity. Patients are able to confront challenges and make decisions about which technology helps them remain motivated to observe their progress.

The principle behind developing tools applied to health is to generate predictions about health states and anticipate possible relapses of disease. The goal is to keep patients and their diseases stable for as long as possible based on personalized data and in real time, leading to a consequent decrease in hospital readmissions.

Turning data into knowledge will not only help to improve the patient experience, but will also enable us to act from the early stages of the health continuum. In this way, artificial intelligence allows for the analysis, interpretation, and prediction future scenarios that help prevent and reduce the burden of chronic diseases. This can also prevent and reduce the impact of diseases on society while improving the general health of the entire population.

Chapter 10

Lifestyle of the Future

10.1 Overview

How are we going to dress in the future? What cars are we going to drive? What will our houses look like? We are not alien to evolution. We can still experience change and adapt to the environment. However, humans are the only species that enhances the process of evolution and adaptation with implants and genetic adjustments.

In the 1970s, scientist Paul Ehrlich predicted that hundreds of millions of people would starve to death despite all the programs that had been proposed to avoid such a crisis. Today, various conjectures have changed our way of life within a few years.

In the 1930s and 1940s, the World Health Organization (WHO), invited people to smoke a cigarette during Thanksgiving dinner as a digestive. Can you imagine how reviled that practice would be today? Life and, in particular, technology can change drastically in a short period of time.

Some studies focusing on the future anticipate more inhabitants and the need for more space. We may wonder whether these studies have accounted for a possible population reduction in the future. Japan is the first country with the greatest decrease in population with 974,000 fewer inhabitants today than in 2010. In the coming years, food consumption habits will need to adapt to new lifestyles where time and practicality will become increasingly fundamental.

Food must be available at any time and place, be practical to ingest quickly, and ensure that needs are met without losing its quality and nutritional properties. This should be done with flexible, simple, and intelligent solutions that facilitate the population's day-to-day lives. Trends show an increase in healthy snacks, with choices depending on specific consumer conditions (vegan, celiac, low calorie, and so on). In turn, packaging will be smaller, appropriately portioned, and designed for consumption on the go.

The concept of convenience also necessitates creativity and incorporates other aspects such as personal health and stories about love, authenticity, and memorable experiences of consumption, for example. Today, there is a greater awareness of health itself, which draws consumers to seek personal care and bet on an individualized diet. These diets are constructed with healthy products and adapted to individual needs. Consumer demand for allergen-free, vegetarian, vegan, and flexitarian options continues to increase.

Likewise, there is increasing demand for environmentally sustainable products that do not involve social or animal abuse at any point. In addition, concepts of proximity, seasonality, and transparency are becoming more important. Increasingly, original and local products are becoming sources of value. Everything seems to indicate that we are on our way to a greater supply of convenient products that are easily adaptable to our personal needs and healthy life objectives.

10.2 Foods We Will Eat in the Future

Have you ever wondered what people will eat in the future? With the technological advances on the horizon, it is probable that in the future, food will change a great deal. Imagine being able to create food that does not have any ingredients. It comes directly from nature or changes color; all sorts of strange innovations are only a few years away.

10.2.1 Meat Created in the Laboratory

On the one hand, the concept might seem appalling, but on the other, proponents of these technologies argue that with a single cell, scientists can create food for the world's population. But is there a scarcity of food around the world? Not really. The supply is just poorly distributed. There is no need for those regenerative cells. There is enough meat for everyone. The general population just can't afford it. For those who are advocates of a meatless life, this is even worse.

10.2.2 Food of Africa

Even though Chinese or Indian food may be trending, the future favorite food will be of African origins. In recent years, a middle class has emerged in Africa, which is likely to be responsible for expanding its culture to other regions. Food is one of the greatest cultural expressions.

10.2.3 Insects

A large percentage of the world's population already consumes insects. Yet many people balk at the idea of insects soon becoming part of one's everyday diet. Insects are rich in protein and low in fat.

10.2.4 Black Bread

Refining flour is an extra job that leaves the flour without essential vitamins. Black bread will become more common in the future.

10.2.5 Encapsulated Fruit

Fruit capsules will allow for the vitamins provided by fruit in the convenience of a small object. Although initially they are going to be very expensive, they will become popular over time and use the advanced machinery available to give them a desirable flavor.

10.2.6 Modified Sugar and Salt

A new variety of salt will be added to meals which will make them healthier. Something similar will happen with sugar. Foods will stop having such large concentrations of sugar.

10.2.7 Verdolaga

This small plant is currently considered a pest, but it will become extremely important in the future. It has high concentrations of beta-carotene and omega-3, both of which are very healthy, and it also tastes good in salads.

10.2.8 Cobia

The cobia is a fish that is bred in fish farms, and it has become one of the integral foods of the future. Due to its adaptive and reproductive abilities, it could become one of the main sources of food.

With the close relationship between cardiovascular health and food in mind, this future development in food sources and materials can have a great impact on creating better cardiovascular health in the future.

10.3 Future of the Fitness World

People seek to take care of their bodies with good nutrition and exercises that allow them to maintain a good state of health. The fitness trend is cashing in on this desire.

Spain and other European countries have introduced interactive gyms. The floors and walls of these gyms cause the machines to recede into the background. With lights, music, and interactive displays, those using the facility are able to become completely immersed in an experience that makes their fitness routines enjoyable.

According to experts, this technological aid will motivate people to exercise. Ending the myth that exercise is boring and stopping users from saying "I can't" is the key to promoting fitness.

These program facilities require people to go through several levels of preparation. The advance with achievement and users are eased into a routine that is suitable for them.

Physical trainers will continue to function as guides for those exercising. This method in Spain and England has resulted in some positive surprises; for example, some people have reported burning up to 750 calories in only five minutes.

10.4 Technology in Exercise

Social networks have initiated these interactive features in the fitness world. People share their routines with others, and the knowledge spreads when followers accept the responsibility to take care of their own bodies. In just a few years, smartphones have become an indispensable tool for work, communication, information, entertainment, and exercise for most of us.

This is a paradigmatic example of technology adoption, demonstrating the extent to which our daily lives can be affected by scientific and technical advances. Health is probably one of the fields that will experience the greatest change in the near future. The possibility to monitor different physiological variables through wearables will open up a promising field of new methods to maintain physical fitness and health and to allow for the early detection of diseases.

10.5 Activation Bracelets and Heart Rate

The famous Fitbit bracelets allow you to keep a record of your physical activity, distance, calories burned, stairs climbed, heart rate, and quality of sleep. The bracelets are synchronized wirelessly with our mobile phones and computers to save a long-term record and allow different applications to take advantage of the stored data. As these devices, like smart watches, incorporate new sensors able to measure things such as body temperature, blood glucose levels, hormones, and changes in sweat, they will become true guardians of our health, capable of telling us when something is not right or giving us advice based on our physiological states.

10.6 Smart Clothes

If the bracelets and smart watches are promising, intelligent clothes could be groundbreaking. Prototypes already exist for T-shirts capable of detecting epilepsy or performing electrocardiograms as well as fasteners for premature detection of breast cancer, or baby bodysuits that change color if the child has a fever. The possibilities are enormous, and hopefully in the coming years we will see a real explosion of clothing with almost magical properties, combining new fabrics with sensors and miniaturized electronic circuits. Recently, I had the opportunity to try out a muscular electrostimulation suit. This was able to provide complete muscular training within twenty minutes once or twice a week, and I cannot help but wonder how long it will be until we see this type of technology incorporated into sportswear controlled by our mobile devices.

10.7 Home Automation

Advances in home automation or technology applied in our home that provides energy management, security, wellness, and communication services, may also have a niche for health, including humidity and temperature control and detection of hazardous and harmful substances or allergens in the environment.

10.8 Feeding

It is a fact that the general population is eating worse. The proportion of overweight and obese people continues to increase across all countries, regardless of culture. At the same time, feeding a growing number of people is a technological and ecological challenge.

Nutritional supplements and sports nutrition have been with us for many years, but it has only been recently that products such as Soylent in the United States and Joylent in Europe have appeared. These products are able to substitute for one or more normal meals. They are not meant to be used on a permanent basis, but there are those who have experimented with living only on these powdered shakes for a month with less surprising results.

While it is unlikely that such products are the future of food, they can be a step toward achieving a healthier, balanced, economical, and environmentally friendly diet. At the moment, they are an interesting alternative while we try to reeducate people on the habits of eating.

10.9 Video Game Consoles

Traditionally enemies of physical exercise, video games have become an unlikely partner in a healthy lifestyle by developing games in which people use their bodies instead of controllers. Systems like the Nintendo Wii and the Xbox Kinect allow users to engage in physical activity in the comfort of their homes in an interactive, motivational, and fun way.

There are also advances such as HoloLens, Microsoft's incredible holographic-augmented reality glasses, or Icaros, a device capable of fusing virtual reality and physical exercise. With these and others, there are infinite possibilities of such technologies in the fields of exercise and physical training.

10.10 Other Devices

Other devices such as electric bikes with greater autonomy and better characteristics, devices to improve and measure sexual performance, prosthetics made with 3D printers and the latest generation materials, and applications for specific smartphones to manage our workouts are also in development.

The possibilities of technology, physical exercise, and health are enormous, with many of them still in their infancy. We are experiencing a kind of Cambrian explosion in this area, and we still have many things to see. Technological advances are happening today with greater speed than ever before in the history of humanity. Many fields are evolving at the same time, and their advances are linked, making the changes bigger, broader, and more all encompassing.

Chapter 11

The Future Starts Now: Be Part of It

11.1 Overview

The treatment of cardiovascular diseases requires patients to modify certain habits and behaviors recognized as risk factors. This is why even with the astonishing developments in pharmacological resources as well as their diversification and optimization, and improved pharmacodynamics profiles and bioavailability, there is no substitute for patients who voluntarily and consciously commit to their treatment.

To remain healthy, it is vital that patients regularly engage in physical activities and eat healthy diets. Most importantly, it is a patient's responsibility to stay up to date on relevant medical conditions. With worlds of information available at our fingertips, it is easier than ever to learn about the dangerous diseases that can affect you and your family. If we pay enough attention to prevention strategies rather than waiting until problems arise, we could avoid tragedy.

The future of CV health is in the hands of both patients and the medical profession. Take ownership of your own health. Take part in informational sessions so that you may become aware of medically relevant topics. Prevention is much easier than treatment. Although you should visit your doctor if you feel something is medically wrong, with the information you have gathered, you will not have to solely rely on his or her diagnosis. You can avoid a misdiagnosis by discussing alternate outcomes.

Make yourself aware of the technological equipment available to you. Teach yourself about the advantages and disadvantages of the technological devices available. Which are the best? How can you use them to prevent future diseases?

Future of Cardiovascular Health

You can join an online CV health community with similar objectives. Find the answers to your questions and help others. These communities will allow you to learn and share new information that can be of help to many others. Sometimes online communities include medical professionals who provide advice about a particular medical situation. This advice comes free of charge.

Find out which hospitals and physicians are best for you. There are various websites or online communities that can assist you in your search. The future of CV health is at your fingertips. Know it, make it, and be part of it.

Glossary

bimolecular: Consisting of or involving two molecules (p. 1).

deterioration: The process of becoming progressively worse (p. 6).

electrostimulation: Electrical muscle stimulation (EMS), also known as neuromuscular electrical stimulation (NMES) or electromyostimulation, is the elicitation of muscle contraction using electric impulses (p. 4).

enzyme: A substance produced by a living organism that acts as a catalyst to bring about a specific biochemical reaction (p. 2).

epidemiology: The branch of medicine that deals with the incidence, distribution, and possible control of diseases and other factors relating to health (p. 1).

holograms: Three-dimensional images formed by the interference of light beams from a laser or other coherent light source (p. 1).

orthomolecular: In complementary medicine, denoting or relating to a form of treatment that seeks to achieve an optimal biochemical balance in the body, typically by the use of large doses of supplementary vitamins and minerals (p. 1).

paradigmatic: Of or denoting the relationship between a set of linguistic items that form mutually exclusive choices in particular syntactic roles (p. 3).

proponent: A person who advocates a theory, proposal, or course of action (p. 2).

transgenic: Relating to or denoting an organism that contains genetic material into which DNA from an unrelated organism has been artificially introduced (p. 5).

vulnerability: The quality or state of being exposed to the possibility of being attacked or harmed, either physically or emotionally (p. 1).

References

Brunetti, Natale Daniele. 2015. "Telemedicine for Cardiovascular Disease Continuum: A Position Paper from the Italian Society of Cardiology Working Group on Telecardiology and Informatics." http://www.telemedico.it/wp-content/uploads/2016/01/position-paper-gruppo-di-lavoro-sic-telecardiologia-e-informatica.pdf.

Centers for Disease Control and Prevention (CDC) State Heart Disease and Stroke Prevention Programs. 2011. Paul Coverdell National Acute Stroke Registry. http://www.cdc.gov/dhdsp/programs/stroke_registry.htm. Accessed September 12, 2011.

Fornell, Dave. 2015. Cardiovascular Advances to Watch in the Next Decade, https://www.dicardiology.com/article/cardiovascular-advances-watch-next-decade

Fornell, Dave. 2017. The Future of Cardiology: 17 Technologies to Watch https://www.dicardiology.com/content/blogs/future-cardiology-17-technologies-watch

Frasure-Smith, N., and F. Lesperance. 2008. "Depression and Anxiety as Predictors of 2-Year Cardiac Events in Patients with Stable Coronary Artery Disease." *Arch Gen Psychiatry* 65: 62–71.

Holm, K. 2010. "Promoting Cardiovascular healthHealth. Special Considerations for the Elderly." *J Cardiovasc Nurs* 25 (3): 252–53.

Huffman, J. C., F. A. Smith, M. A. Blais, et al. 2008. "Anxiety, Independent of Depressive Symptoms, Is Associated with In-Hospital Cardiac Complications after Acute Myocardial Infarction." *J Psychosom Res* 65: 557–63.

Kaczorowski, J., L. W. Chambers, L. Dolovich, et al. 2011. "Improving Cardiovascular Health at Population Level: 39 Community Cluster Randomised Trial of Cardiovascular Health Awareness Program (CHAP)." *BMJ* 342:d442.

Kruse, Clemens S., Mounica Soma, Deepthi Pulluri, Naga T. Nemali, and Matthew Brooks. 2017. "The Effectiveness of Telemedicine in the Management of Chronic Heart Disease—a Systematic Review." https://www.ncbi.nlm.nih.gov/pmc/articles/PMC5347273/.

Salisbury, Chris. 2016. "Telehealth for Patients at High Risk of Cardiovascular Disease: Pragmatic Randomised Controlled Trial." Retrieved from http://www.bmj.com/content/353/bmj.i2647.

Santamore, W. P., C. Homko, J. Marble, J. Wald, A. A. Bove. 2004. "Improving Heart Failure Care by Using a Telemedicine System." https://www.ncbi.nlm.nih.gov/pubmed/17270928.

Schwamm, Lee H. 2017. "Recommendations for the Implementation of Telehealth in Cardiovascular and Stroke Care." http://circ.ahajournals.org/content/circulationaha/early/2016/12/20/CIR.0000000000000475.full.pdf.

Wade, Victoria. 2017. "The Use of Telehealth to Reduce Inequalities in Cardiovascular Outcomes in Australia and New Zealand: A Critical Review."

http://www.heartlungcirc.org/article/S1443-9506(16)31687-0/pdf.

WHO Library Cataloguing-in-Publication. 2010. "Data Telemedicine: Opportunities and Developments in Member States: Report on the Second Global Survey on eHealth 2009." http://www.who.int/goe/publications/goe_telemedicine_2010.pdf.

Wong, Crystal. 2017. "AHA Recommendations for Telehealth in Cardiovascular and Stroke Care." http://www.thecardiologyadvisor.com/stroke/cv-and-stroke-care-telehealth-rrecommendations/article/632811/.

Thank You